Get Through

**Clinical Finals:
A Toolkit for OSCEs**

Get Through
Clinical Finals:
A Toolkit for OSCEs

Andrew Papanikitas BSc (Hons) MA MBBS
Senior House Officer
Aylesbury General Practice Vocational Training Scheme

Nawal Bahal BSc (Hons) MBBS
Senior House Officer
Anaesthetics and ITU, Oldchurch Hospital, Romford

Michelle Chan BSc (Hons) MBBS
Senior House Officer in Ophthalmology
Royal Free Hospital, London

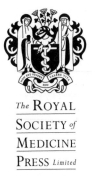

The ROYAL
SOCIETY of
MEDICINE
PRESS Limited

British Library Cataloguing in Publication Data
A catalogue record for this book is available from the British Library

ISBN 1-85315-615-9

Distribution in Europe and Rest of World:
Marston Book Services Ltd
PO Box 269
Abingdon
Oxon OX14 4YN, UK
Tel: +44 (0)1235 465500
Fax: +44 (0)1235 465555
Email: direct.order@marston.co.uk

Distribution in the USA and Canada:
Royal Society of Medicine Press Ltd
c/o BookMasters Inc
30 Amberwood Parkway
Ashland, OH 44805, USA
Tel: +1 800 247 6553/+1 800 266 5564
Fax: +1 419 281 6883
Email: orders@bookmasters.com

Distribution in Australia and New Zealand:
Elsevier Australia
30–52 Smidmore Street
Marrikville NSW 2204, Australia
Tel: +61 2 9517 8999
Fax: +61 2 9517 2249
Email: service@elsevier.com.au

Typeset by Phoenix Photosetting, Chatham, Kent
Printed and bound by Replika Press Pvt Ltd, India

Contents

Part 5 Special situations

Part 6 Practical skills

Preface

There's no getting away from the fact that finals are *tricky*. Not difficult but tricky, like riding a bike or swimming. Once you know how to do it, it is second nature, but before you do, it can be akin to a miracle.

Many people will tell you how unfair finals can be, about how they got a distinction in the written only to fail the clinical exam. The truth is that no other exam reflects adequate preparation better than the clinical finals.

Our aim when preparing for the finals was to be ready for 'the googly', to use a cricketing term. The result was a comprehensive list of what we expected, how to approach it, and how to shine. We also realized just how useful what we learned could be to future students. Not just a checklist of things to do but things not to do, and how to assess what is wanted of you.

There exists an obscure area between being a final-year medical student and becoming a confident House Officer. It involves possessing and implementing an understanding of not only medicine, surgery and psychiatry but also ethics, communication and administrative skills, amongst others. This book is intended to help identify this whole area and show the reader the common pitfalls and, by combining such information, how to successfully 'mind that gap'.

Nawal Bahal
Andrew Papanikitas
Michelle Chan

Acknowledgements

We would like to thank our parents for support and encouragement, as well as Miss Andrea Ogden, Miss Niran Bahal and Miss Victoria Hyslop. We would also like to thank the staff of the Conquest Hospital, Hastings, including Dr Richard Wray, Dr James Dennison, Dr Martin Clee, Mr Simon Baer, Mrs Lesley Rudling, Miss Nikki George, as well as Mr Niall Aston, of Queen Elizabeth Hospital, Woolwich for an honest practice OSCE; and Dr Joseph Papanikitas, Dr Richard Freeman, Dr Toby Gillman and Dr Taryn Youngstein for test-driving the manuscript.

We are indebted to the following for the sometimes harsh but fair peer-review including Kai Keen Shiu, Giles Kendall, Kin Yee Shiu, Maxine Tran, Sarita Singh, Arani Nitkunan, Tarek Maani, Litha Pepas, Suparna Das, Krishnan Venkataraman, Martin Paul and Clementine Maddock.

Finally, we would like to thank Professor Ronald Marks, Cardiff, for providing the dermatology pictures and Mr Bob Tapper for the ophthalmology photos. We are indebted to Alison Campbell and Hannah Wessely at the RSM Press for their patience and hard work in developing our manuscript.

Nawal Bahal
Andrew Papanikitas
Michelle Chan

Part 1

Basic framework

1 Introduction

How to pass your medical finals

This chapter is primarily aimed at finalists at the beginning of the final year. Bad advice is stated as **bold quotes** so you can avoid these pitfalls early. We state the obvious, because we were amazed at how many really obvious advantages we missed when starting to prepare for exams.

'There is no advantage in finding out what came up in previous years.'

This FALSE statement is based on two incorrect premises:

- The first is that the OSCEs are sufficiently different each year to make previous knowledge worthless. While this can be true, OSCEs take an astonishingly long time to develop and a very large amount of criticism before they are removed from the exam.
- The second premise is that knowing what is in the exam confers no advantage. While it is certainly true that candidates knowing exactly what is on the mark sheet are not guaranteed to get 100%, it is also the case that good preparation is difficult without knowledge of previous OSCEs. Once you have an idea of what has come up before, you can use those formats to design your own OSCEs. Just remember that there is always a first time for things to come up so it is best to revise as much as possible from all clinical years.

Find out why you passed and/or failed previous OSCEs. Feedback should also be available from your previous years, though you may need to persevere to get it. It is worth sitting down and trying to work out what happened. Be honest. Did you pass because you deserved to? Were you lucky? Did knowledge get you through, or are you naturally good at OSCEs? Beware of thinking this, as *savoir-faire* is more likely to desert you on the day than good practice and preparation.

'Revision involves guessing what will come up and ignoring everything that seems non-core. The following subjects are a waste of time: ethics, communication skills, public health, evidence-based medicine...'

Every year finalists come out of written exams and OSCEs ashen-faced, muttering things like 'So much public health... What was that ethics question about? What was I supposed to do in that OSCE station?'. Ignore the above subjects at your peril and avoid the trap of not knowing enough clinical medicine, surgery, pharmacology, etc. See our chapters on public health, ethics and communication skills for some ideas on how to approach this.

'Accept no criticism and ignore advice from people who have just qualified.'

A certain number of people cannot understand why they failed and come out of exams thinking that they have passed when in fact they have not. Hints, tips, advice and even past papers are often dutifully filed away and never again seen. If you feel you have been given bad advice or unconstructive criticism then check with colleagues or another senior. People who have just qualified may be very busy but most are happy to divulge the content of their exams (see end) and how to tailor what you have learned to OSCEs and life on the wards. Passing finals comfortably is rarely a solitary effort. The start of the final year demonstrated to the authors that though we had been taught a great many useful things, we had learned very few of them!

'To revise for finals, you clearly need to find the biggest textbook you can and read it from cover to cover. Practice questions and group work are for losers.'

The key to revision is practice questions – a chapter a day keeps resits at bay! Revision guides, the *Oxford Handbook of Clinical Medicine* (Longmore et al, OUP) or *Clinical Medicine*, Student Edition, (Kumar and Clark, Elsevier) are the way forward. Stay away from big books! The best practice question books are the ones that explain the answers. The gold standards at the moment are (MCQs) *Clinical Medicine: Key Questions Answered* (Wai-Ching Leung, OUP; (EMQs) *EMQs for Medical Students, Vols 1 and 2*, (Feather et al, Pastest); and for a glimpse of how hard, easy, cruel and bizarre final-year questions can be, *Get Through Medical School* (Coales and Khan, RSM Press), is a good way to acclimatize to SBA and BOF questions and EMQs.

'If you are having problems with a placement, there is no point doing anything about it.'

What might be wrong with a placement? An insistence that students take part and know their stuff is hard to criticize, especially if it includes clinical experience and teaching by the team. However, lack of supervision, patient exposure and relevant clinical experience are frequent causes of anxiety. Staff are too busy, patients in too much discomfort. It sometimes seems that if most qualified doctors had their way, medical school would be one long 'go for a coffee...' Remember that:

- There are many opportunities to be taught and see patients with relevant histories and signs, but you have to ASK and organize a 'learning round'.
- Even the worst placement can be made good if you get together with other students and do a daily student teaching/learning/mock OSCE round.
- If a placement is irremediable, all teaching hospitals have a subdean who you can talk to (sooner rather than later). Clinical advisors or course organizers should be approached if this fails.
- You may have the nicest team in the world but don't get trapped on the world's longest business round if it means missing teaching or missing seeing a patient with signs who will shortly be cured, discharged, etc.

'Work alone, you are in competition with your peers.'

Working with others allows you to pool knowledge, to test and practise on one another (within the limits of decency). Role playing and testing one another's knowledge in the presence of others is the only way you can find out your weaknesses and turn them around. Bear in mind that 'everyone hates a sponge'. If you are the least able member of a group and your role-playing skills are abysmal, find some way of contributing, even if it is as the coffee boy/girl and examination dummy. Similarly, if someone is using your group as a glorified coffee morning then something must be said. Sometimes a revision can get too big as students migrate along a teaching/learning gradient in the approach to finals. Secrecy is one answer. Meiosis into smaller groups, perhaps working in the same area but rotating between stations, is a nicer way of doing things.

'Revision plans take too long and are a feature of obsessive-compulsive disorder – don't bother with them.'

If you work to a plan you will get through everything. One way is to take every type of station and timetable the last three weeks, including weekends and some evenings. Allow for tutorials and some ward time and *keep to the plan*. The plan will only succeed if it is worked out with achievable targets and is really only suited to those who can fully commit their time. Cover everything.

Don't leave structured and time-pressured learning until the last minute, because the skills lab and tutorial rooms will rapidly fill with people more motivated than you or, worse, less motivated people desperate to find someone who will carry them through exams.

In the last week before the exam

'In the written, do the exam as quickly as you can and then leave early.'

Though traditional SAQs, essays and even MCQs have been replaced by best-of-five questions and extended matching questions, it is never worth leaving before the exam is over. The idea that you will spend the last few minutes changing correct answers to incorrect ones is largely a myth. Check that you have actually answered the question. Beware of questions containing the words 'never', 'always' and 'not'. These should be read carefully. Practice questions are useful, even in the last week.

'In the last week there is nothing you can improve on. Ignore any weaknesses and hope for the best.'

This is another myth! Even with 24 hours to go, a new skill can be learned.

In the OSCE

ALWAYS read the instructions outside a station. These often effectively tell you what the marks are for and you do not have time to do anything other than what you are instructed to do. If an examiner interferes, 99% of the time they are trying to help. Never argue with an examiner, this is a waste of time.

Don't take the exam too seriously

It is worth remembering that exam nerves are a significant cause of exam failure. The other thing to remember is that there can be mistakes in the exam, sometimes astonishing ones. Bells go off in the wrong place, examiners think they have a break and you find a patient but no examiner, stations make no sense, external examiners get in the way, rests are strangely positioned and you miss them, Asian men in their early 20s turn out to be 65-year-old ex-smokers called Stan, and you may discuss the teratogenic effects of warfarin with a lady well past child-bearing age. Take exam preparation seriously but try to relax on the day.

If you think a station has gone badly, forget about it and move on

This is easily said but very hard to do. There can also be a temptation to write off a station *while you are in there*. This is fatal. It is true that you can compensate in other stations but always try to stay engaged and focused on the station you are in. You can score points right up until the end.

Courtesy and empathy score points

Many OSCE stations invite the patient or actor to rate your performance, and have marks allocated for how you interact with a patient in terms of courtesy, empathy, etc. If you are confident enough not to care about these points, remember that they could make the difference between fail and pass or pass and prize.

Après ski…

After the OSCE, it is always worth noting what came up and what was easy and what was hard (and why). This is for two reasons:

- There's that slim chance (hopefully now slimmer) that you or a friend will be resitting.
- A House Officer who can advise his or her students on finals is a popular House Officer.

General approach to the OSCE exam

Four things you need to know about OSCEs

1. They test core knowledge and skills. That means no 'small print' or rare conditions but does not mean that the smaller subspecialties such as ENT, dermatology or ophthalmology should be omitted.
2. They test minimum competence. During your preparation, keep reflecting on your performance. Am I confident enough with my examination? Do I struggle with the questions in history taking? The ultimate acid test is: Do I look or sound like a doctor?
3. Most students fail their finals because they fail their OSCEs.
4. OSCEs are easy to pass and easy to fail. They are easy to pass because they ultimately examine the things that you already know as a final-year student, assuming you have done a reasonable amount of work. OSCEs are also easy to fail by committing fatal errors, such as:

- being unsafe
- looking unsure throughout the exam
- not knowing what to expect (do you know how many marks you will lose by simply forgetting to introduce yourself in each station?)

How to plan your OSCE revision

Find out the facts about your exam

It is vital to know the structure of your exam. How many OSCE stations are there? How much time is allocated to each station? What is the spread among history taking/examination/explanation/skills?

Past OSCE questions

Ask the students from the years above which stations they were given. A significant amount of repetition is likely because OSCEs test core knowledge and skills. Were there any unexpected questions? The chances are you will also get some similarly unexpected questions, so be prepared.

Plan your revision time

How you spend your OSCE revision time depends on where your strengths and weaknesses lie and how the marks for the exam are distributed.

Divide the preparation into manageable chunks

Be realistic and write an outline of 'chunks' of material to include everything you need to prepare for. The point is to admit to yourself how much work needs to be done and to make a plan for yourself. Make each chunk a mix of history, exam and skills, something that can be tackled in a single revision session.

Simulate OSCE conditions

The best practice is to simulate a real OSCE as closely as you can. Always time yourself. Do not allow yourself to stop half way to ask questions or make fun of the situation. Be as careful and methodical as you would during the exam itself. Use the correct instruments – tendon hammer, stethoscope, ophthalmoscope. Borrow some tools if you can to practise at home – dressing pack, suture packs, neuropins, urinary catheter, Venflons, etc. Practise with another student; examine your family members.

Tackle your demons

It is important to know what you *don't* know. So before you start revising, be honest and write down:

- key topics you have avoided preparing all along
- key topics you have some idea of but are not comfortable with
- less important topics you are not familiar with (usually the smaller subspecialties).

Spend some time tackling these topics first. Get them out of the way and you'll find the revision getting easier.

Pass as many stations as you can

Remember, your aim is to **pass** as many stations as possible, not perform brilliantly in a select few. It is dangerous to skip topics in your revision or only focus on physical examination at the peril of ignoring the explanation and communication stations.

Part 2

Skills in communication and ethics

2 Communication skills

Scorned by medical practitioners and overlooked by students since time immemorial, the importance of effective communication in medical practice is now beginning to be appreciated. To a certain extent, communication is assessed at almost every station in finals. Mastering these skills is important. Reading about them is not enough; they need to be *practised*.

In most OSCEs you will be given a vignette before seeing the patient, so you will often know what is about to happen (i.e. telling someone they have inoperable cancer of the lung). It is important to be calm and impartial. Do not get ahead of yourself either; many a student has fallen on their sword by telling a patient with a suspected cancer of the bowel that 'Dukes' A has a good prognosis' when all the patient wanted to know was whether she could drive home after her colonoscopy! Exploring patient's ideas, concerns and expectations (Table 2.1), open questions, effective use of silence, giving the patient options are all weapons in your armory.

Breaking bad news

- Introduce yourself to the patient.
- Ask if anyone is with them. Would they like them present?

TABLE 2.1 ICE – ideas, concerns, expectations

All actors have these and so do all patients

- Ideas – 'What do you think this has been caused by?'
- Concerns – 'Are you worried that this may be due to anything in particular?'
- Expectations – 'What do you expect from us?'

- *Switch off your bleep and/or make sure you will not be disturbed.*
- Recap what has occurred so far.
- Offer a warning shot. 'Your test results have now come back but it wasn't the result we'd hoped for' or 'I'm afraid it isn't good news'.
- Break the bad news. Come out with it, don't pussyfoot around. If you are unclear, the patient becomes uncertain and the agony is prolonged.

Do not forget to pause. Allow bad news to sink in. The patient may want to voice a question or concern.

Your next comment might be 'Do you understand what I've just told you?' or 'I realize I have given you a lot to think about. Is there anything you would like to ask me?'.

For Example:
What might a patient want to know about the following diagnoses?

- Multiple sclerosis
- Epilepsy
- Rheumatoid arthritis
- Ankylosing spondylitis
- Myasthenia gravis

Invite questions and answer them as simply as you can. Five questions that you should be prepared to answer about a diagnosis are:

- Will I die?
- Is there a cure?
- Will I have to give up my work or the things I enjoy?
- Will I pass this on to my children?
- Will I be paralysed?

Ways of letting the patient know that they have support

- Offer written material in the form of information booklets, websites and telephone numbers for support groups.
- Invite the patient to return at any time if they or their friends/relatives have any questions.
- Make the patient aware that you will see them again.
- Offer your bleep number if they wish to contact you directly.
- Thank the patient and say goodbye.

If you don't know the answer to a question, do not lie. Admit you do not know, apologize and tell the patient you will find the answer (for example) from a senior colleague and let them know before they leave.

Explaining/negotiating

More often than not, there is an element of negotiation involved as well. Hear the patient out and deal with their beliefs appropriately.

- Introduce yourself and recap what has occurred so far.
- Remembering *ICE*, explain to the patient what needs to be done. 'This sounds like a viral infection and the best way to manage this would be to take paracetamol and plenty of fluids for the next week.' Allow them to express their views.
- Discuss the pros and cons of two separate methods, e.g. action (surgery and cure) versus waiting (no intervention, no cure), or antibiotics (cost and side-effects) versus supportive management.
- Reach a management decision, showing respect for the patient's autonomy.
- Sum up what you've discussed.
- If relevant, offer some written material, e.g. for colonoscopy/ERCP.
- Offer further support and keep the option of further meetings open.
- Thank the patient and say goodbye.

Important points for particular situations

- Stay calm if the patient gets upset.
- Some stations require a review of relevant data. For example, with hypertension management, enquire about smoking, alcohol, exercise, stress, diet, blood pressure.

*Techniques for dealing with aggression**

Defuse the aggression by acknowledging what the person is saying or doing and then moving on to solutions.

- 'I can see you are angry/worried/upset. Is that because…?'
- 'You don't like the way I handled this situation. What would you like me to do?'
- 'You are unhappy about this. Do you have any suggestions as to what I should do about it?'

You may need to interrupt the other person.

- 'I'm not happy with this, please stop.'
- 'The way you are talking is not acceptable to me.'

*Houghton A. Tips on… Dealing with bullies. *BMJ Careers* 2005; May 14: 201.

If your time is up and you are getting nowhere (should not happen in the OSCE!):

- 'I'm going to leave now. Let's talk about this when you are feeling calmer'.

Cross-cultural stations – some examples to practise

1. You are called to see the father of a young man who has died from a head injury. He is a practising Jew and would like the body to be released for burial, untampered with (see Chapter 4).
   - Express your condolence, and state that there is a further matter that needs to be discussed (you are essentially breaking more bad news).
   - Explain that an autopsy is needed. In this case the medical team has no say in the matter, as it is required by law.
   - Explain what an autopsy is and why it is done.
   - The Coroner *orders* an autopsy, he or she does not *request* one. The family has no legal right to stop one going ahead.
   - You can try and make sure the autopsy is performed as a priority so the burial can occur within 24 hours of the death, in keeping with Jewish custom.
   - Offer to contact the hospital rabbi if desired.

2. You are called to speak to an irate woman on the ward. Her lesbian partner is an inpatient and they have both been receiving verbal abuse from other patients on the ward. She would like her partner moved to the side room (which you know is occupied by a very ill leukaemic patient).
   - Listen to the complaint of verbal abuse against the patient due to her sexual orientation (complaint made by partner against other patients on ward).
   - Come up with a mutually agreeable solution (official complaint/move to different ward/inform sister and nurses to be on lookout for abuse/inform all patients of hospital policy against all forms of abuse).
   - Negotiate a compromise.
   - Remember that confidentiality must be respected; you should not divulge details about the patient in the side room to a third party.

3. The patient who speaks a foreign language. Remember that this OSCE tests your *ability to communicate,* rather than your knowledge of what constitutes best practice in terms of informed consent. Though you should assess and comment on the appropriateness of an interpreter (particularly family members who may have their own agendas), the emphasis is on all the different verbal and non-verbal stratagems that you employ (Figure 2.1).

This is a real skill but easily practised with friends. A patient will attend who cannot speak English. The medical condition is usually obvious and not serious. The patient will often have an agenda of their own, such as a desire to obtain antibiotics for a viral sore throat.

- Introduce yourself.
- Take patient's name and assess level of English.
- Establish where they are from and what language they speak.
- Ask if someone is with them and, if appropriate, do they speak good English?
- State that you would request an interpreter to be present or would ask whether there is anyone in the department/practice who speaks the language.
- Point to yourself and say 'I am Dr Smith'. Then point to the patient in an enquiring way.
- Use pen and paper if provided to write your age and then invite patient to do the same (most cultures use Arabic numerals).
- 'Problem?' Point to parts of your body.
- Say 'Ow!' to signify discomfort and wait for patient to agree (head, throat, chest).
- Signify vomiting, diarrhoea, shivering and sweating.
- Timing – use a calendar if available, otherwise *write* the date and *say* the day.
- Manage the problem (usually a question of whether antibiotics are needed).
- Check that the patient understands what to do.
- Write down instructions for an English-speaking friend of the patient to translate for them.
- Thank the patient and say goodbye.

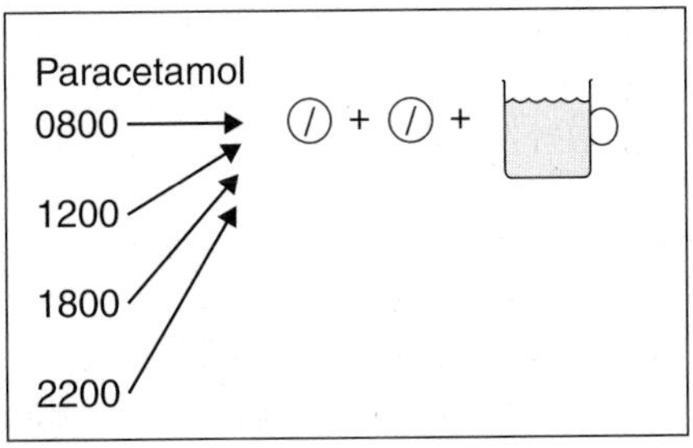

FIGURE 2.1 Regimen for paracetamol for a viral infection for someone who does not speak English. This is easy to draw, if pen and paper are available.

Remember:

- Do not patronize the patient.
- Do not raise your voice.
- Do not take on the patient's accent when you repeat what they say.
- You are being assessed on your non-verbal communication skills. Do not start a conversation in 'Greek' with a 'Greek' patient, as you will get no points for this, and the actor probably speaks no 'Greek' anyway!

The astute medical student will be aware that asking some people to translate may violate confidentiality, especially when asking family members, friends or employers to act as translators. Use common sense. Written instructions for the treatment of a viral throat infection are hardly in the same category as a prescription for the 'morning-after pill'.

4. You are the GP PRHO. Mr Syed Ali (a 24-year-old newly diagnosed diabetic) has come to see the GP because, although he is an insulin-dependent diabetic, he is also a devout Muslim and would like to fast during the season of Ramadan.

   - Find out from the patient what his religious practice involves and to what extent he is prepared to comply with treatment. Does he wish to abstain from food and drink or is he keen to omit his medication as well?
   - Also establish what treatment he is on. Is this working? What does he know about his illness? Does he test his own blood sugars? Is he willing to learn how to do this? If he intends to fast then this may be necessary.
   - Are others around him aware that he has diabetes? Would they know what to do in the event of a hypoglycaemic episode ('hypo')?
   - Explain that although asymptomatic while well controlled, diabetes is an illness and hypoglycaemia can rapidly become life-threatening. Therefore the patient could be forgiven for carrying sugar in some form with him in case of a 'hypo' or warning others about the signs of a hypoglycaemic episode.
   - His insulin regimen can be modified but he can make things easier by altering his eating habits, for example having 'slow-burn' foods (i.e. a proper meal) before dawn and after dusk, rather than the fatty and sugary high-calorie snacks that are traditional. He needs to avoid wide variations in his blood sugar. This can be discussed at length with the practice nurse/diabetes team and you should reassure him that the team will support him during this period.
   - There is an NHS leaflet, 'Diabetes in Ramadan', to give to the patient, who may also benefit from introduction to other Muslims with the condition. You can offer to discuss this further with family members or a religious representative, if the patient would consider this helpful.

- *Do not presume* to lecture the patient on the theology of Ramadan, even if you have an academic or personal knowledge (the actor is not necessarily a Muslim). The point is to negotiate with the patient based on the patient's ideas, concerns and expectations.

Interprofessional relationships

This involves having to discuss an issue with another member of staff, usually not a doctor. They are often quite stubborn, occasionally rude. Let them have their say, but avoid colluding with a colleague or patient against another colleague or patient.

The idea is to reach a mutually acceptable management decision.

1. A nurse has somehow offended or mishandled a patient, who is threatening to complain.
   - Be non-judgmental.
   - Find out what happened.
   - Offer to explain what happened to the patient and, if necessary, discuss the patient with other more senior ward staff together.
   - Ask the nurse if they can speak to the patient later or whether they would prefer you saw the patient together.

2. A radiographer refuses to do an urgent investigation after hours.
   - Allow the radiographer to voice their grievance (within reason). They may dislike your team and say so.
   - Apologize for your team's previous behaviour (see 'dealing with aggression' above).
   - Gently remind the radiographer that regardless of the team, the patient's interest comes first.
   - Come to a mutually agreeable decision.
   - Always leave a bleep number and ask to be informed of the result of any urgent investigation.
   - The station might also involve filling out a form or pointing out that it is incomplete or incorrect.

3. Your Senior House Officer needs time off to study for MRCP, arrange a mortgage or have a nervous breakdown, and wants you to carry his bleep for the day.
   - Despite what may seem common practice, you are **not** supposed to say yes.
   - Find out why he wants to be away. Be supportive. This station is usually supposed to last seven whole minutes!

- Offer alternatives. You could ask the nurses to bleep you in preference, and he could delegate anything that you are capable of handling. He could hand his bleep to another SHO. Has he discussed the need for some time off with a consultant or registrar?
- Remember that there are some things you need a senior for – e.g. advice, 'do not resuscitate' orders, prescription of streptokinase, etc.

4. You have noticed a colleague making a dangerous prescription error. You corrected it in time but this is not the first dangerous mistake you have prevented. Please talk to your colleague before taking any further action.
   - Ensure some privacy and open the conversation in a general manner: 'How have things been over the last few weeks? How have you been coping with the job.'
   - Be as non-judgmental as possible, but bring up the specific incidents.
   - Find out, if possible, if there is anything you can do to help or anything that your colleague can do to help himself.
   - Come to a mutually agreeable decision about this if possible.
   - You may need to gently remind an uncooperative colleague that if you are convinced that he is putting patients' welfare in danger, you have a duty to speak to someone (you do – see GMC *Duties of a Doctor* in Chapter 3).

3 Ethics for OSCEs

Is it all common sense?

Many people assume that ethics is all common sense, and that this applies especially to exams and naturally to OSCEs. Unfortunately, common sense can sometimes turn out to be unethical or illegal.

OSCE scenarios fall into three types of case: those that can be argued either way (where those preclinical lectures come in handy!); those where there is a clear professional (ethical) duty to do (or not do) something; and those where you are under clear legal obligations.

Ethics for OSCEs is more than four words

Ethics is taught at medical school in terms of four principles:

1. **Beneficence** (do good)
2. **Non-maleficence** (try not to harm)
3. **Autonomy** (you give information and options but the patient chooses)
4. **Justice** (is what you are doing fair?).

These four principles might be useful in thinking about a scenario where you have to weigh pros and cons but they are not all that useful when you are discussing a case in an OSCE. A good knowledge of the relevant ethical and legal duties is comparatively priceless.

Hint: It is a good idea to try to attend ethics symposia, debates and lectures because many scenarios that come up here may end up in exams in some form or other. Make a special effort to attend *anything* involving *actors*, because these scenarios are more likely to be recycled in clinical exams. A scenario is always easier to deal with if you have thought about the issues already. In the unlikely event that you have never attended anything involving ethics or communication, at the very least look at the GMC's *Duties of a Doctor* (see below) and think of some plausible situations in which you might find them challenged or conflicting. You can try role playing these and similar scenarios with colleagues. Ideally, work in groups of three or four (one role-player, one student, one timer/marker).

Example scenarios

Scenario 1

You go to see your clinical advisor, because your consultant has had a complaint made against him by a patient. In front of you, he told the patient, using a popular expression, that she had very attractive breasts. He is denying this and wants you to act as his witness before the GMC. He has yet to write your report/reference.

What you are expected to do

Reason through this. Is the answer as simple as it sounds? To obtain full marks, you need to discuss the pros and cons of your actions, the consequences for you, the consequences for him and the consequences for the patient.

If you are a truthful witness, the pros are that you have carried out your professional and ethical duty. You have done nothing 'wrong'. However, you have put a highly skilled and possibly essential person in danger of being reprimanded for professional misconduct. He will certainly not be writing your reference. He may accuse you of lying and you may acquire a reputation as a whistleblower.

If you tell your consultant that you cannot act as his witness, as you would be obliged to tell the truth as you remember it, then you do not prejudice his career and perhaps save yours, but the patient may suffer the injustice of being called a liar. Perhaps if he apologizes to the patient the proceedings may be dropped.

Lying is always the wrong answer. Here, you would be effectively stating that you would violate a patient's dignity to cover up a colleague's professional misconduct. But then again, a simple statement that you would report him will not get you many marks either. This one can be argued more than one way.

Scenario 2

After much probing, a patient finally tells you that he has become HIV positive, but he does not want this to appear in his notes because he is in the process of renewing his life insurance and is worried that it may affect his work (he is an operating-theatre nurse).

What you are expected to do

Reason through this. Is the answer as complicated as it sounds? You need to negotiate what you can and cannot do for the patient, in order to obtain full marks. If the patient is prepared to tell his dentist and other carers, your obligation to enter the information into the notes is not absolute *unless* you think he will knowingly put others in jeopardy. Then you have a professional duty to write something or tell someone (and to *sensitively* tell the patient this). HIV status is not a question insurance companies can insist on but must be left blank and not falsified.

Again, lying is always the wrong answer. However, this man may need to get a new job and this needs to be *sensitively* negotiated.

Scenario 3

A newly diagnosed epileptic bus driver clearly has no intention of informing the Driver and Vehicle Licensing Authority, and does not want his condition recorded in the notes.

This is relatively clear. You have a legal and professional duty to him and to the public. Driving will place both in considerable danger. However, you need to be able to explain this and explore options such as other skills or retraining. He will lose his PSV licence (for at least 10 years) in any case but he may be allowed to drive himself after a year 'fit free' on medication. If he remains adamant that he will not inform the DVLA, you must tell him, sensitively, of your duty to do so.*

---

*A guide to common illnesses and the duty to inform the DVLA can be found on page 162 of the *Oxford Handbook of Clinical Medicine*, Longmore M, Wilkinson I, Rajaqopalan S, Oxford University Press, 2004.

Ethics comes into most things

The following situations all involve an assessment of your duties and responsibilities: discharging a patient following a surgical procedure or acute medical condition; establishing informed consent for a test or procedure; counselling a patient on their risk for a sexually transmitted disease; negotiating with a colleague who is not coping and wants you to take unauthorized responsibilities or has had a mishap involving a patient; and even dealing with complaints.

Conscientious objection

In today's multicultural society, doctors do have a right of conscientious objection, i.e. they do not have to do things that are against their conscience or religion, but a life-threatening situation *always* supercedes this and where an objection does hold, there is still a *legal duty to refer to another doctor*, especially where contraception and abortion are concerned.

Potential sources of medicolegal conflict often arise as a result of religion in clinical practice, as the following examples show:

- Is circumcision mutilation? The UK law says that it is for girls but not for boys. Benefit must be weighed against harm, and courts routinely take decisions out of the hands of parents, especially where one parent says 'yes' and the other parent says 'no'.
- Is there a legal duty to take part in abortions? Theoretically, no one should have to perform an abortion or sign the relevant form against their will. There is a conscience clause in the Abortion Act but it only affects those directly involved. There is a legal obligation for doctors to refer to another practitioner. A legal duty to perform an abortion may exist irrespective of conscience if a woman's life is in danger.
- Should a Jehovah's Witness be forced to receive blood in their own interests? The law respects the autonomy of a competent individual. This does not include children. *An adult's previous advance refusal is legally binding.* This can include a card stating that a person has an advance refusal to particular treatment.

Never (and this does actually happen) tell a patient that they are 'evil' or attempt to use religious arguments to dissuade them from action or inaction. This applies even if the patient is of the same faith as you. To do this is widely viewed as inappropriate, especially in an OSCE. The concept is not as silly as it sounds, as there are many cases where a patient's religious observances may lead them to refuse treatment (the Jehovah's Witness undergoing major surgery, the diabetic Muslim in Ramadan).

In all cases, you are supposed to be non-directive, i.e. finding out what a patient's religion means to him or her, before providing relevant options or advice (and herein lie the marks). Remember that in an OSCE, an actor's grasp of a religious concept and yours may be very different. We have never heard of a candidate going so far as to try and evangelize an OSCE patient, though when a student attempted to evangelize a real patient, this resulted in disciplinary action. Standing in judgement over any patient, real or false, is also obviously inappropriate.

Duties of a doctor, according to the GMC (read this at the very least)

The text in brackets are some suggestions of where these duties might be challenged.

- Make the care of your patient your first concern (*even if the patient is intending to do something reckless or to harm others or is threatening you?*)
- Treat every patient politely and considerately (*even if the patient is uncooperative, does not speak English or is verbally abusive?*)
- Respect patients' dignity and privacy (*even if their religion dictates that they cannot have life-saving treatment or insists on treatment widely viewed as mutilation, or if their privacy or dignity means risking harm to another?*)
- Listen to patients and respect their views (*even if their beliefs are not based on scientific fact, are bizarre or just plain wrong?*)
- Give patients information in a way they can understand.
- Respect the rights of patients to be fully involved in decisions about their care (*even if the patient is stupid, mentally handicapped or ill, senile or a minor?*)
- Keep your professional skills and knowledge up to date.
- Recognize the limits of your professional competence (*even if modesty might cost you a good job? What if a senior needs you to cover for them in an emergency?*)
- Be honest and trustworthy (*will honesty get you into trouble?*)
- Respect and protect confidential information (*do you give an insurance company all information about your patient, or all relevant information, even if they have asked for the former?*)

- Make sure your personal beliefs do not prejudice your patients' care (*even if you believe that referring a patient to another doctor is just as bad where your religious beliefs are concerned?*)
- Act quickly to protect patients from risk if you have good reason to believe that you or a colleague may not be fit to practise (*will this end a friend's career? Will this potentially end yours?*)
- Avoid abusing your position as a doctor.
- Work with colleagues in ways that best serve patients' interests (*can you think of any circumstance where a doctor might be tempted to conflict with this?*)

In all these matters you must never discriminate unfairly against your patients or colleagues. And you must always be prepared to justify your decisions to them.

The OSCE frequently calls on us to justify our actions, and life even more so. If you want to do the right thing and be able to justify it, then forewarned is forearmed. The above section should start you thinking along the right lines.

4 Obtaining consent for a post mortem

Obtaining consent for a post mortem (PM) or, more often, breaking the news to relatives that a coroner post mortem will be necessary is often part of the final-year OSCE. This is something that needs to be dealt with *sensitively*. As with any other communication scenario, you should explore what the next of kin know and whether they have any questions *before* you launch in with a potentially devastating request.

- A post mortem is a careful and respectful internal examination of the body.
- It is carried out by a pathologist assisted by a qualified technician.
- It is conducted to standards set down by the Royal College of Pathologists, including carrying it out in a respectful manner.
- There may be appreciable benefits: the PM may exclude a contagious or inherited problem or set relatives' minds at rest as to the cause of death.
- It may still leave some questions unanswered.

A **Coroner PM** is ordered in the case of a sudden or unexpected death, where the cause is unknown and a death certificate cannot be issued, or if the cause is other than natural disease, e.g. occupational disease such as mesothelioma.

Deaths should be referred to the Coroner in the following circumstances.*

- The cause is unknown.
- The practitioner has not attended the deceased during their last illness.
- The practitioner neither attended the deceased during the last 14 days before death nor saw the body after death.

*Branthwaite M, Beresford I. *Law for Doctors*, 2nd edn. RSM Press, 2003, Ch 9.

- Death occurred during an operation or before recovery from the effects of an anaesthetic.
- Death was caused by industrial disease or poisoning.
- Any death believed to be unnatural or caused by violence, neglect or abortion.

The above cases are discussed with the Coroner. They are independent of the hospital and only the timing of the autopsy is negotiable. *'The Coroner issues the death certificate and contacts you to let you know when to proceed with funeral arrangements.'*

It is particularly important to treat a Coroner PM as a 'breaking bad news' scenario (See Chapter 2 on breaking bad news): *'Unfortunately none of us have any choice in the matter. This is something which the Coroner orders and is required by law.'*

Common pitfall: a very definite faux pas with a Coroner PM is to use the word 'we', as in 'We need to do an autopsy so that we can find out why your son/daughter/mother died'. This can set up an 'us and you' relationship, which is unhelpful.

A **consented (hospital)** PM is requested if a more detailed diagnosis is sought. It may help others with the same disease and may avoid finding out too late about other problems in other family members. This does not delay the issuing of a death certificate and *does* require consent from the next of kin.

'How soon is the post mortem conducted?'

As soon as possible, within 2–3 working days. If religious observances require it to be done within 24 hours then every effort is made. *This can be a negotiable point.* Some tests on organs or samples take weeks. The next of kin needs to know if this might delay a funeral. *'On the form you can state whether you agree to organs being retained for further tests or research, and how you wish them dealt with after the PM.'*

'Will the body be disfigured?'

In most cases marks on the body and head will not be noticeable as they will be covered by clothes and by the hairline. Sometimes the pathologist can go through existing surgical scars.

'What is done?' (This is something that should be asked about rather than volunteered)

The pathologist carries out an external examination and takes photos and x-rays for detailed study. A cut is made down the front of the body and internal organs removed for detailed examination. Samples or parts of organs may need to be removed.

DEATH CERTIFICATE

You may issue a death certificate* if:

- You have seen the patient alive within two weeks of death.
- You are satisfied that death was due to natural causes.
- You are reasonably sure of the cause of death.
- Death does not require referral to the Coroner.
- You have the appropriate form: Medical certification of cause of death.

When filling in the form:

- Avoid abbreviations.
- Part 1a is the disease or pathological process directly leading to death, e.g. bronchopneumonia (not asphyxia).
- Parts 1b and 1c are diseases underlying this, e.g. chronic obstructive pulmonary disease.
- Part 2 includes any diseases that may have contributed to death but not directly as in Part 1, such as ischaemic heart disease in the above case.
- Complete both the certificate and the counterfoil.
- The 'Residence' is your professional (hospital) address.

Some hospitals have a highly developed bereavement service; others rely on you to hand the certificate to the relatives in a sealed envelope with the 'notice to the informant'.

*Morrit AN, Hall J. Completing a death certificate. *BMJ Careers* 2004: May 328:217.

5 Perioperative advice

These OSCE stations primarily revolve around the patient's ideas, concerns and expectations

- Ask if they know which anaesthetic they are to have.
- Take a very quick history, e.g. of ischaemic heart disease or respiratory problems.
- Elicit any family history of operative complications, especially personal/ family reactions to anaesthetic.

Example: Preparation for laparoscopic surgery

- No food for six hours before.
- Clear fluids until two hours before.
- Drip will prevent dehydration.
- May have bowel prep (admit on preceding day).
- The patient will meet the surgeon who will obtain consent and be able to answer more specific questions.
- The patient will meet the anaesthetist and discuss need for pre-med (midazolam).

When the patient wakes, they may have:

- oxygen mask on
- a catheter and lines inserted
- a Voltarol (diclofenac) suppository
- patient-controlled analgesia (morphine with cyclizine); tell relatives not to press button while patient sleeps and not to use mobile phones.

Laparoscopic surgery always carries the (small) risk of conversion to open surgery, with the consequence of a wound and a scar.

The patient may go home when:

- they are physiologically well
- they are walking
- pain is controlled (regional anaesthesia may still be working; patient should be advised to take provided analgesia when instructed to prevent painful interval between feeling pain and tablets working).

The patient must be:

- picked up in a car
- going to a home with a phone
- less than one hour from the hospital
- with someone to look after them for 24 hours.

They may take home:

- paracetamol or a stronger analgesic
- other drugs (depending on operation).

A follow-up letter will be sent to the GP. Stitches may be removed in the GP surgery, at a clinic or by the District Nurse. If wound care is required, the District Nurse often provides this.

Lifestyle advice

- No driving or operating heavy machinery for 48 hours after a general anaesthetic.
- Only drive after insurance company has been contacted, the patient is pain free and is comfortable performing an emergency stop.
- Following surgery such as a hernia repair, avoid a rise in intra-abdominal pressure (no heavy lifting, control coughing and avoid constipation). Prostatic symptoms may be relevant.
- Varicose veins: patients wear thromboembolic-deterrent stockings (TEDS) for a certain period and tight stockings for a further period.

Example: Spinal versus epidural anaesthesia

- Spinal anaesthesia normally done at L3–L4 (midway between the iliac crests).
- Epidural anaesthesia is done T_5–T_{12} or L_1 to L_5.

- Spinal anaesthesia is a single injection below the spinal cord (cord terminates around L1) and there is a smaller risk of infection than with the indwelling catheter for an epidural.
- Spinal offers a heavier block than epidural, allowing more painful surgery.
- Both last 3–6 hours but epidurals can be topped up.
- Both may cause a significant drop in blood pressure.
- Both can be used in conjunction with a general anaesthetic.
- Epidurals can be used if patient-controlled analgesia will be insufficient for postoperative pain relief.
- Patient is normally sat up during insertion of spinal/epidural.

Tell the patient:

- to expect numbness and paralysis
- that local anaesthetic is given before a spinal, therefore they should only feel a small needle
- that they will be catheterized (because of urinary incontinence), normally after the anaesthetic is given.

Complications

- The needle may hit blood vessels and nerves.
- Infection.
- BP drop. If there is a postoperative BP drop it is not necessarily due to the anaesthesia; if there is no change to the epidural and the patient's BP drops, it is probably due to another cause.

Local blocks

This is regional, e.g. an ileo-inguinal block is sometimes used for a hernia repair (1 cm medial and below the anterior superior iliac spine).

Choice of anaesthetic

- Poor respiratory function makes a general anaesthetic less likely.
- Fixed cardiac output states (e.g. aortic stenosis) mean NO SPINAL.

Preoperative information (these are things that appear on OSCE mark sheets)

Do you elicit the patient's concerns?

- Being awake in theatre.
- Being alone.
- Pain.
- Nausea.

Do you explain the anaesthetic procedure?

- Preoperative medications.
- Someone will remain with them throughout.
- A screen will be up to prevent the patient seeing the operation.
- The patient should only feel a small needle (sharp scratch).
- Numbness lasts for hours afterwards if having spinal/epidural.
- If there are problems, may go from local anaesthetic to general anaesthetic.

POSTOPERATIVE PAIN RELIEF

- IM/IV opiates.
- Suppositories (these need special permission for use).
- Oral medications.
- Management of nausea.

Part 3

History and counselling skills

6 History taking

You will not be able to take a history during an OSCE as fully as you would in real life. Instead, aim to elicit a condensed version with fewer details but all the appropriate headings nevertheless. The history should:

- be relatively brief
- cover the 'key features' – every symptom has its key features. A cough with weight loss and haemoptysis is more worrying than a nocturnal cough which only occurs in the spring
- cover the standard areas – all histories should include presenting complaint, past medical history, drug history and allergies, family and social history
- try to start with open questions, then narrow your focus.

How to take a history effectively

1. Brief simple greeting: 'Hello, I'm Jane Smith and I'm one of the doctors here'.
2. Reflect the information already given; do not waste time asking them again.
   - Set the scene: 'I understand you're in A&E because of chest pain...'
   - Establish the general picture: '...and that you had a heart attack two years ago...'
   - Then get the patient to talk: '...so can you tell me about the pain you are getting now?'
3. Spend the bulk of the time on the presenting complaint. However, in some cases, the past history is just as important, such as previous cardiac events and investigations in a patient with chest pain.

4. Functional history:
   - Whatever the disease or condition, do not forget to ask how it affects the patient's daily life, work, independence and emotional well-being, e.g. exercise tolerance in patients with chest pain and breathlessness.
   - Activities of daily living for patients with chronic diseases.
   - For a patient in chronic pain, is the pain affecting their sleep or mood?
   - 'Is there anything else I should know?'
5. Aim to spend some time summarizing and encouraging questions near the end of the station, probably when the final warning (usually one minute) is given.

How to take a history professionally

Aim to be polite and personable, sympathetic and tactful. Make the history sound like a conversation, not an interrogation.

1. Be polite. Greet the patient. Be tactful if you need to interrupt: 'I'm sorry, but can we just go back to...'
2. Be personable. Smile, if appropriate, and maintain eye contact.
3. Be sympathetic and tactful: 'I'm sorry. This must be very difficult'. If the history has touched upon an upsetting or difficult situation, the worst thing to do is to ignore it. If a patient/actor cries, stop the history/examination and check if they are all right and allow some silence.
4. Make the history flow:
   - Phrase your questions as an invitation to the patient to talk: 'Why don't you tell me about...'
   - Acknowledge the patient's answers: 'yes', 'right' 'I see'.
   - You could be checking off a list of questions in your head but, to make the history sound natural, change the subject smoothly. 'So, apart from the chest pains and heart problems we have just talked about, do you have any other medical problems?' 'Now that we've been through your medical history, I need to ask you a few routine questions about yourself. What do you do as a living? Where do you live?', etc.

The art of focused history taking

Taking a focused surgical history

This station usually involves an actor and an examiner, who will give you examination findings and test results, *usually only when you ask for them.* (See taking a medical history below.)

Introduction

● Hello, my name is John Smith; I'm one of the doctors. Can I ask you your name?

Presenting complaint and history of presenting complaint, including relevant questions about pain, and relevant system (e.g. abdominal) questions

● What's the problem? When did it start? Is there any pain?
● Where is your pain exactly? Have you had this pain before?
● How did it begin? How bad is it now?
● Is it aching, burning, stabbing, crushing, squeezing? Does it come and go in waves?
● Does the pain go anywhere (does it radiate)?
● Has it become worse, better or stayed the same? How long has it lasted?
● Does anything make it better or worse? Does any position make it better or worse? Have you taken any medicines for it and did they help? Are you having any other problems (vomiting)?

A common scenario is some form of **acute abdomen**:

● Appendicitis, constipation (or any cause of large bowel obstruction), ruptured ectopic pregnancy (a differential not to be missed).
● Adhesions, obstructed or strangulating hernia (any cause of small bowel obstruction).
● Peptic ulcer, leaking abdominal aortic aneurysm, acute pancreatitis

'Is there any chance whatsoever that you might be pregnant? Have you had sex in the last few months?'

Any woman of child-bearing age with pain in either iliac fossa may have an ectopic pregnancy. *This is life threatening and must be excluded.*

Remember that any woman of vaguely reproductive years who presents with abdominal pain or per vaginal bleeding needs a menstrual history, a brief sexual/contraceptive history (the IUD and progesterone-only pill may be associated with ectopic pregnancy) and a pregnancy test. Ectopic pregnancy is a differential diagnosis for appendicitis, amongst other things.

Always ask **relevant focused questions** first. Then move on to the following:

● Previous medical/surgical history
● Are you taking any medicines at the moment? Anything unprescribed?
● Do you smoke and – this is confidential and we need to know – do you take any street drugs?

- Do you drink any alcohol? What do you usually drink? How much do you drink in the course of a week?
- A social history scores points. Is there anyone the patient would like to call? Is there anyone waiting with them? Are they elderly or disabled, living in a house or flat, are they doing a job that needs to be curtailed temporarily or permanently?

Ideas, concerns and expectations (these count!)

- Is there anything in particular that you are worried about?
- Is there anything in particular that you would like to know?

Summary

- Think what history questions and examination findings might give clues.
- Think what the appropriate investigations might be.
- Think whether the patient needs to go straight to theatre or have a specific investigation.
- Senior review is mandatory.
- Always discuss the next stages of management with the patient.

To revise for this station, find a book that details relevant investigations and differentials, e.g. *Surgery at a Glance,* 3rd edition, Grace P and Borley N, Blackwell Science, 2006.

Taking a focused medical history

Focused history taking for medicine is similar to that for surgery. The variety of conditions and differentials in undergraduate finals is greater, however. As with psychiatry, it is useful to think in terms of differentials, e.g. is a loss of consciousness neurological, syncopal or metabolic?

> **'This patient presents to A&E with an episode of syncope. Take a history and suggest the relevant next steps in management.'**

Screen for causes of syncope. Marks come mainly from advice: need to admit for further tests (primarily to exclude dangerous or common pathology), appropriate referral to specialist, advice on long-term medication, driving, work, etc. Ask relevant history, diagnose, then discuss treatment, referral, etc.

For any diagnosis, think:

- what is the most dangerous differential (and how do you exclude it)?
- what is the most likely differential?

Some other examples…

- Nausea, vomiting, altered consciousness: DKA? Food poisoning?
- Altered consciousness following a fit: postictal, hypo- or hyperglycaemia?
- Chronic shortness of breath on exertion in an elderly man: cardiac or respiratory?
- Joint pain: infective arthritis or rheumatological condition?
- Chest pain: cardiac, pulmonary embolus, respiratory or musculoskeletal?
- Acute shortness of breath: asthma, angina, pneumothorax, pulmonary embolus?
- Back pain: always ask about constant pain, night pain and thoracic pain (these are 'red flag' symptoms needing investigation).

7

Specific histories

Cardiac and respiratory histories

Chest pain

If the pain is suggestive of cardiac origins, elicit symptoms of cardiac failure, assess functional ability and elicit cardiac risk factors.

In known ischaemic heart disease, how often does the patient get angina? Have they had an MI? Have they had an exercise test, radionuclide scans, angiogram, angioplasty or bypass surgery?

- Onset: at rest/exercise induced?
- Duration, site, character, severity, radiation?
- How quickly does it wear off?
- Alleviating and aggravating factors?
- Breathlessness, dizziness, palpitations?
- Previous episodes and frequency?
- Exercise tolerance?
- Able to lie flat? How many pillows at night? Swollen ankles?
- Previous cardiac history, investigations and treatments?
- Cardiac risk factors: smoking, diabetes, hypertension, hypercholesterolaemia, positive family history?

Breathlessness

First of all, is the cause cardiac – ischaemic/arrhythmic/pulmonary oedema? Or is this respiratory? If so, is it infective?

TABLE 7.1   Causes of chest pain

Cause	Characteristics
Acute coronary syndrome (angina, MI)	Crushing, heavy central chest pain May radiate to left arm or jaw Exercise induced Breathlessness, dizziness Nausea and vomiting if severe
Arrhythmia (e.g. fast AF)	Palpitations – awareness of heartbeat
Musculoskeletal pain	Sharp pain, movement induced, previous history of muscle strain. Localized tenderness
Oesophageal pain	*Very similar to cardiac pain* May be precipitated by food
Pleuritic chest pain	Sharp pain worse on inspiration

Functional assessment is important: what can the patient normally do? How far could they walk before? And how is it different now?

In known COPD/asthma patients, how often do they experience an exacerbation and what triggers it (cold air, exercise, chest infection, stress)? What treatment do they use at home – inhalers, oral steroids, nebulizers, oxygen? In their previous admission, how long did they stay, did they need ITU admission?

- Onset: at rest/exercise induced?
- Duration, severity?
- Cough and sputum: amount, colour, smell?
- Fever?
- Chest pain: pleuritic/central crushing?
- Dizziness, palpitations?
- Previous episodes and frequency?
- Exercise tolerance?
- Able to lie flat? How many pillows at night?
- Paroxysmal nocturnal dyspnoea?
- 'Do you ever wake up in the middle of the night feeling breathless?'
- Smoking history: cigarettes/roll-ups, amount/day, number of years?
- Known COPD: ambulatory oxygen, previous admissions and treatment?
- Known asthmatic: frequency of inhaler use, previous admissions and treatment?

Palpitations

Palpitation means something different to everyone, but it usually refers to a strong awareness of the patient's heartbeat. Do they show signs of cardiac ischaemia? Did it cause syncope?

TABLE 7.2   Causes of breathlessness

Cause	Characteristics
COPD exacerbation	Long-term smoker, poor exercise tolerance
Pulmonary oedema	Inability to lie flat, >2 pillows at night, swollen ankles, paroxysmal nocturnal dyspnoea
	Cardiac history
Asthma exacerbation	Induced by: exercise, dust, cold air, stress, NSAIDS, a specific allergen
	Cough
Chest infection	Fever, cough, yellow-green (i.e. coloured) sputum

- What exactly did you feel?
- Were you very aware of your heartbeat?
- Was it fast/slow? Regular/irregular? 'Can you tap the rhythm?'
- Breathlessness?
- Chest pain?
- Faint and dizzy, collapse, loss of consciousness?
- Previous episodes?

Gastrointestinal histories

Abdominal pain

- Onset, duration, site, severity, radiation, character?
- Vomiting, Haematemesis?
- Relationship to bowel action?
- Diarrhoea?
- Rectal bleeding?
- Weight loss?
- Urine and menstrual history (pregnancy?) can be relevant

Obstruction: colicky pain, vomiting.
Infective: colicky pain, vomiting, diarrhoea, fever.
Acute appendicitis: starts in mid abdomen, migrates to right iliac fossa.
Acute cholecystitis: right upper quadrant pain (can radiate to the shoulder tip), vomiting, jaundice.
Acute pancreatitis: epigastric pain, radiates to back.
Inflammatory bowel disease: fever, vomiting, recurrent diarrhoea, weight loss.

Vomiting

- Onset, frequency?
- Vomitus: amount, contents (especially blood), colour, smell?
- Nausea?
- Abdominal pain?
- Diarrhoea?
- Headache?
- Jaundice?

Diarrhoea

- Acute or chronic?
- Normal bowel habit: frequency, consistency, colour?
- Current bowel habit?
- Frequency?
- Stool:
  - amount, colour, consistency, loose, watery?
  - bulky, smelly, difficult to flush away – steatorrhoea?
- Blood or mucus:
  - mixed in with the stool?
  - on top of it?
- Infective cause:
  - abdominal pain?
  - vomiting?
  - fever?
  - foreign travel?
  - other people infected?
- Non-GI cause:
  - drugs: antibiotics?
  - thyrotoxicosis?
- Symptoms of malignancy:
  - weight loss?
  - blood in stool?
  - previous episodes of constipation?
  - family history?

Constipation

- Bowel habits: frequency, effort (need to strain)?

- Stools:
  - consistency, amount?
  - blood: mixed in or on toilet pan?
  - anal pain?
- Symptoms of malignancy:
  - is there a change of bowel habit?
  - weight loss?
  - tenesmus?
  - family history?
- Symptoms of obstruction:
  - abdominal pain?
  - vomiting?
- Precipitants:
  - hydration and diet?
  - hospitalization, lack of privacy?
  - opioids?

Rectal bleeding

- Onset?
- Blood:
  - amount?
  - fresh/dark?
  - mixed in with stool/on toilet pan/only on paper?
- Pain on defaecation?
- Constipation?
- Symptoms of malignancy:
  - change in bowel habit?
  - tenesmus?
  - weight loss?
  - family history?
- Infective: vomiting, diarrhoea, fever, abdominal cramp?

Haematemesis

- Preceding symptoms (sharp pain and vomiting: Mallory–Weiss tear)?
- Frequency and amount?
- Colour of blood:
  - fresh (varices, Mallory–Weiss tear)?
  - coffee grounds (gastric/duodenal ulcer)?

- Abdominal pain?
- Symptoms of shock: dizzy, faint, breathlessness, chest pain?
- Alcohol history/drug history/NSAIDs?

Dysphagia

The main differential is between a mechanical cause and a motility disorder. It is also important to elicit features of an oesophageal malignancy.

- What happens? Food get stuck? Regurgitation?
- Solids/liquid?
- Is it difficult to initiate the swallowing?
- Pain on swallowing: odynophagia?
- Does this happen all the time or only intermittently?
- Weight loss?

Jaundice

- Duration?
- Intermittent, coincides with other illness (Gilbert's Syndrome)?
- Colour of stool and urine?
- Abdominal pain? (gallstones?)
- Alcohol abuse?
- Drug history?
- Hepatitis risk:
  - IV drug use?
  - foreign travel?
  - blood transfusion?
  - sexual history?

Neurological histories

Headache

For headaches, the basic details of onset, duration, site, character are the most important and are diagnostic.

- Signs of serious causes: seizures, impaired consciousness, meningism (neck stiffness)?
- Onset, duration, site, character, severity?

- Precipitating and alleviating factors?
  Visual disturbances:
    - colourful zigzag lines or blurred vision?
    - before or after the headache?
    - transient or constant?
    - photophobia, phonophobia?
- Vomiting?
- Seizures?
- Loss of consciousness?
- Neck stiffness?
- Fever?
- Skin rash?
- Functional history: loss of sleep, depression, poor concentration?

TABLE 7.3 Causes of headache

Cause	Characteristics
Tension headache	Gradual onset at the end of day
	Like a band around head
Migraine	Unilateral throbbing headache – usually over one eye
	May be preceded by visual aura that disappears after the episode
	Photophobia, phonophobia
	Lasts for hours/days
Raised intracranial pressure	Early morning severe headache
	Associated vomiting
	Constant blurred vision
Subarachnoid haemorrhage	Sudden, severe, 'thunderclap' headache with collapse
	May be loss of consciousness and seizures
	Neck stiffness afterwards
Meningitis	Gradual severe headache
	Fever, vomiting, neck stiffness
	Petechial rash – meningococcal sepsis
	May be associated seizures

Blackout/'funny turn'

A witness is often needed to clarify the facts of the event but the patient's account of how they *felt* and what they *remembered* is also very important.

- Onset:
    - 'What exactly were you doing before you blacked out?'
    - 'What was the last thing you remember before blacking out?'
- Loss of consciousness?
    - 'Were you rousable? Could you hear people calling you?'

- Before the attack:
  - dizziness/hot: simple faint?
  - severe headache, vomiting, neck stiffness: neurosurgical cause?
  - prodromal symptoms, *déjà vu*: epileptic seizure?
  - chest pain/palpitations/breathlessness: cardiac cause?
- During the attack (witness account):
  - did the patient change colour?
  - twitching or jerking of limbs?
  - incontinence of urine or faeces?
  - duration of attack?
- After the attack:
  - 'Do you remember waking up?'
  - 'How did you feel after you woke up?'
  - 'Drowsy? Wet trousers? Tongue bleeding, cuts and bruises?'
- Prior head injury, alcohol and drug use?
- Previous episodes and frequency?

TABLE 7.4   Causes of blackout/funny turns

Cause	Characteristics
Syncope	Feeling dizzy, nauseous, sweaty beforehand
	Provoked by emotion, pain, fear, heat
	Regains consciousness rapidly
Epileptic seizure	Prodromal symptoms – aura, *déjà vu*, hunger
	Identifiable precipitant – TV, strobe light, hypoglycaemia
	Generalized or focal jerking of limbs
	Loss of consciousness for seconds to minutes
	Postictal drowsiness
Transient ischaemic attack	Sudden onset
(vertebrobasilar territory)	Impaired consciousness for <24 hours
	Associated focal neurology
Stokes–Adams attack	Transient brachycardia due to complete heartblock
	Pale; slow pulse
	Quick recovery (seconds)
Subarachnoid haemorrhage	Sudden severe 'thunderclap' headache

TABLE 7.5   Causes of collapse without loss of consciousness

Cause	Characteristics
Ischaemic heart disease	Central crushing chest pain, precipitated by exertion
Drop attacks	Sudden weakness of the legs causes the patient to fall to the ground. Full consciousness. No precipitant
Menière's disease	Sudden severe vertigo and vomiting
Benign positional vertigo	Severe vertigo precipitated by head movement
Mechanical fall	Physical impairment, loose carpets, etc.

Rheumatological histories

Functional and social histories can be more significant in rheumatology than in other systems.

Presenting complaint

- Identify all joints affected: upper and lower limbs, neck, hip and back.
- Which joint(s) is the worst? Which symptom is the patient most troubled by?
- Joint pain:
  - onset, duration, site, severity, radiation?
  - differentiate joint and muscle pain?
  - worse at the end of the day, relieved by rest (OA)?
  - precipitating and relieving factors?
  - which joints affected first? Progression?
- Swelling?
- Stiffness: early morning (RA) or worse through the day (OA)?
- Peripheral neuropathies: numbness, tingling, muscle weakness?
- Extra-articular symptoms:
  - weight loss?
  - fever?
  - skin rash: SLE – photosensitivity, butterfly rash; psoriatic plaques – non-itchy scaly patches; poly/dermatomyositis – heliotrope rash on face?
  - cold sensitivity (Raynaud's syndrome)?
  - oral/genital ulcerations (Behçet's disease)?
  - dry mouth and eyes (Sjögren's disease)?
  - red eyes (RA, Reiter's syndrome)?
  - preceding gastroenteritis/urethritis (Reiter's syndrome)?

Functional history

- Loss of function:
  - occupation?
  - hobbies?
  - activities of daily living (mobility, using the toilet, bathing, grooming, feeding, cooking, cleaning)?
- Sleep disturbance?

Abbreviations: OA, osteoarthritis; RA, rheumatoid arthritis; SLE, systemic lupus erythematosus.

Past medical history

- Possible systemic manifestations:
  - anaemia, thrombocytopenia?
  - pulmonary fibrosis, pleural effusions?
  - pericarditis?
  - renal disease?
  - entrapment neuropathies?
- Ask if any previous history such as Crohn's disease, Ulcerative Colitis, Psoriasis?

Drug history

- Drug allergies can cause polyarthritis.
- Analgesia: including side-effects?
- Steroids: oral and injections to joints, including side-effects?
- Immunosuppressants?

Family history

RA and OA can show familial predisposition.

Social history

- Housing and adaptation?
- Loss of independence?
- Social isolation?
- Smoking and alcohol?

8

Psychiatry for OSCEs

As far as last-minute cramming goes for written and OSCE, use a practical handbook not a large reference text book. If somehow you have remembered nothing, playing the game and revising common complaints is a start. Practice questions and scenarios are a must. A tutorial with a registrar or consultant is usually very helpful and this chapter aims to give a similar style of advice.

For the psychiatry OSCE, in a 7½-minute station assume you have six active minutes at most.* Time runs much too fast in these things. Break it up into two minutes for the presenting complaint, two minutes for specifics and two for a summary, diagnosis and management, assuming that some time will be lost in reading instructions and transferring between stations.

> 'Hello, my name is [your name], I am one of the doctors working here. Can I ask you your name? How old are you? What do you do? Why are you here?'

Never forget to introduce yourself and ask:

Name
Age
Occupation
Marital status

During further questions, you are assessing any patient's risk to themselves and others, and getting a good history of presentation and previous illness, as

*Different medical schools allocate different amounts of time, but it never seems enough.

well as asking about obvious risk factors and sequelae, for example, any financial difficulties, job loss, marital difficulty, trouble with the law or physical consequences when taking an alcohol history (as well as CAGE questions – see Box).

Sometimes a surgical approach can be helpful...

Site: What is wrong? (depression/anxiety/psychosis)
Onset: When did you start to feel something wrong?
Character: How does it make you feel? Is there any insight?
Radiation: How is it affecting the other aspects of your life?
Associated factors: Crime? Substance misuse?
Timing: Precipitating factors ('Can you tell me what started this?/What do you think this is due to?')
Exacerbating/relieving factors
Severity

The summary includes whether you feel the patient should be treated as an in/outpatient, what investigations they should have, and what medical or non-medical management is needed. If there's any doubt over the risk, *admit* the patient initially.

A good opening gambit is: 'We've not met before. I wondered if you would tell me what problems you've been having. Did you want to come and see us or did someone bring you?'

Start with open questions and then use closed questions to clarify. 'At this stage I need to know more. When did it start? Did anything set it off? What makes things better or worse? What do you think all this is due to? Have you had any illnesses in the past?'

Favourites for psychiatry stations are suicide, depression, schizophrenia, bipolar disorder and alcohol problems. OSCE exams also tend to use scenarios with a possible differential to exclude or a risk to take account of.

Past psychiatric history may be relevant. If so, ask about previous diagnosis, previous treatment, including admission, medication and compliance. Does the patient have a CPN (community psychiatric nurse)? Is the CPN helpful? Do they keep in contact?

Some questions will be more specific to the presentation: 'Do you have odd experiences that other people do not share? Do you hear or see things that others do not?'. This might distinguish delusional disorder (no hallucinations) from schizophrenia (third-person auditory hallucinations). Are delusions persecutory, grandiose, nihilistic or do they fit a described pattern?

The psychotic patient

The key aim of such a station in an OSCE is to make sure you know the crucial difference between persistent delusional disorder and schizophrenia, which is basically that:

- Schizophrenia is delusions *with* hallucinations (third-person auditory).
- Persistent delusional disorder is delusions *without* hallucinations, or other symptoms such as passivity phenomena.

Persistent delusional disorder has a much better prognosis than schizophrenia. Remember that 'abnormal experiences' may be drug induced. The fact that you do not need hallucinations to have a diagnosis of schizophrenia is one of those 'real-life' things that do not apply in OSCEs. If a patient in an OSCE has schizophrenia, he should have third-person auditory hallucinations.

Delusions divide into:

- persecutory (common)
- grandiose (e.g. special powers)
- nihilistic – dead/dying/rotting/world about to end, etc. These are not metaphors; the patient doesn't *feel* dead, they *are* dead.

Remember the differentials

A 'voice in the head' is not necessarily a hallucination. An hallucination is when a patient believes there is someone talking to them. Second-person auditory hallucinations can be associated with depression and alcoholic hallucinosis but remain common in schizophrenia. Visual hallucinations should make you think of organic brain disease.

What treatment should you suggest?

- Admit in order to begin antipsychotic medication.
- Admit in order to observe medication free.
- Let them go home.

Anxiety

Anxiety disorders can be described as follows:

- Generalized: all the time. No precipitants.
- Panic: not all the time, attacks 'out of the blue'.

- Phobic anxiety: predictable precipitants, even thinking about them may produce symptoms.
- Obsessive-compulsive disorder produces anxiety if the patient cannot act on a compulsion.
- Post traumatic stress disorder (PTSD): look for the triggering event.

First-line treatment is cognitive behavioural therapy, second line is antidepressants, third is anxiolytics.

For PTSD, use questions about ability to relax, intrusive thoughts and memories, exaggerated startle (hypervigilance and hyperarousal). With alcohol abuse, and most other patients, it is worth asking about smoking, street drugs, medications and social circumstances: **'How is this affecting your family? How is this affecting your life?'**.

Depression and its differentials

Depression, when moderate, will display somatic features, which can be used to separate it from an organic problem such as a dementia (is the patient elderly?). Memory and concentration difficulties, especially in the elderly, could be dementia or depressive pseudodementia.

'Do you have trouble sleeping? Do you wake very early in the mornings? Are things not as enjoyable as they used to be? What is your appetite (or libido) like?' are useful screening questions.

Depression in OSCEs is usually of moderate severity with biological symptoms:

- Altered sleep
- Altered libido
- Altered appetite/weight
- Agitation/retardation
- Diurnal variation (worse in the morning)
- Differential diagnoses: organic illness (e.g. hypothyroid), cognitive impairment, psychotic symptoms.

Tailor your questions to the presenting complaint. You need to ask about alcohol (CAGE questions if appropriate) and sometimes about drug use, past or present. *It is critical to ask the patient about thoughts, plans or history of suicide attempts.* Are there any regrets if someone is being counselled after an attempt? A 'para suicide' needs to be asked about: plans, notes and what stopped them. Where suicide is planned but not attempted, a useful question is 'what is stopping you'? This may elicit protective factors.

Remember that CAGE stands for the following:

'Have you ever felt the need to **C**ut down your drinking?'
'Does people's commenting on your drinking **A**nnoy/anger you?'
'Do you ever feel **G**uilty about your drinking?'
'Do you ever need an **E**ye-opener (alcohol) in the mornings?'
A score of *three out of four is significant* and should prompt further questioning.

Depending on the presentation, a depressive-type history may turn into a cognitive state exam. For finals, you must be able to apply the relevant bits of the 30-question mental state exam as found in the *Oxford Handbook of Clinical Medicine.*

What are the words in the briefing?

Forgetfulness?
Poor concentration?
Clumsiness or difficulty with complex tasks?
Does the vignette suggest a mood or memory problem?

The mental state test should be used to ascertain whether there is a problem with attention, concentration (**'Spell "world" forwards then backwards'**), registration, retention or recall? Is the patient orientated? **'What is the day/date/month/year/time of day? Where are we?'** – department, floor, building, city.

Can they retain and recall a plausible address, such as 'Joan Smith, 42 West Street, Dulwich'? Do they remember the name of the Prime Minister or monarch, the capital of France? There is no point in testing drawing and writing unless there is some evidence from the presentation that clumsiness or difficulty with physical tasks is an issue.

The Abbreviated Mental Test Score

1. What month is it?
2. What year is it?
3. Where are you now?
4. Recall this address…
5. Name these three objects…
6. What is your name?
7. Do you remember the date World War I started (1914) or World War II (1939)?
8. Name the current UK monarch.
9. Name the current Prime Minister.
10. Count backwards from 20 to 1 without an error.

General approach to psychiatric stations

- All OSCE stations should really start with open questions, e.g. 'I understand that you have been feeling a little down lately. Can you tell me a little more about that.'
- Past medical history (any illnesses/admissions/treatments) – exams often put in something irrelevant just to make them realistic and to give you a mark for asking
- Alcohol
- Drugs, both prescription and illicit
- Smoking
- How is the problem affecting your family life?
- Make use of silences, avoid turning a psychiatric history into an interrogation.

A word of caution

Sometimes an OSCE patient may be briefed to try to involve you in their delusion. So when you are asked 'How many teabags do you think I stole?', volunteering a figure invites the response 'So you think I stole the teabags as well?'. Similarly, some patients, especially with mania, are very flirtatious, and a certain professional distance needs to be kept for obvious reasons.

There may be marks for *empathy*. Touching the patient is not always appropriate and some say that it is frankly hazardous in a non-examination station. If someone is being quite florid or quite threatening in any way, you can say 'This seems to be making you very angry'. Similarly if someone keeps bursting into tears, 'You do seem to be very upset…'.

Remember

- Introduce yourself.
- Be understanding.
- Do not be too formal – you will just sound out of place.
- Do not expect much coherent interaction from the patient. You might not be able to take the history in an orderly fashion, depending how cooperative or distracted the patient is.

The focus of a psychiatric history

- Tailor your approach to the scenario as there is rarely time to do everything.
- Current complaint.
- Mood.
- Insight (do they know they have a problem?).
- Risk of self-harm.
- Diagnostic features of the condition and differentiation from other psychiatric disorders.
- Past psychiatric history and treatment (see below).
- Drug and alcohol misuse.
- Social situation – marital status, employment, living conditions, support network

At the end, you will be asked to summarize your history, give a diagnosis and perhaps comment on the patient's speech, thought and behaviour. Be prepared to suggest a plan of action.

Practice psychiatry stations and specific questions

Depression

Scenario 1

Craig is a 70-year-old man who has come to speak to his GP because he has been feeling low for some time.

Introduction

'Good afternoon, Craig. I'm Dr Jane Smith. How can I help you?'

Assess depressive symptoms

'How do you feel right now?'

'How would you describe your mood?'

'How long have you been feeling low like this now?'

'Do you feel depressed all day long?' (depressed most of the time but with diurnal variation)

'Is there a particular event that triggered it?' (e.g. bereavement, financial problems, alcoholism)

Assess suicide risk – 'Have you thought of harming yourself?' 'How far did you go with the planning?' 'What stopped you?' 'How do you see yourself in the future?' 'Can you see a time when things will be better?'

Elicit diagnostic symptoms of depression

'Have you noticed a change in your weight and sleep?'
- 'Loss of appetite?'
- 'Weight loss?' 'How much?'
- 'Insomnia?' 'Every night?'
- 'Early morning wakening?'

'Lack of energy?' ('Do you feel tired all the time?')

Poor concentration?

Agitation/retardation? ('Do you feel you get agitated?' 'Or do you feel yourself getting a bit slower?')

'Anhedonia?' ('Have you lost interest in the things you used to enjoy?')

'Feelings of guilt and worthlessness?' ('Do you blame yourself for things that were not your fault?')

Association with other psychiatric disorders?

'Are you seeing or hearing things that other people can't see/hear?' (schizophrenia)

'Have you ever felt very high and excited?' (bipolar disorder)

Past psychiatric history

'Have you seen a doctor about this before?'

'What treatment have you tried (medication, compliance with tablets, counselling, etc.)? Do you find it helps?'

Alcohol, drug and social history

'Do you drink alcohol?' 'How much do you drink?'
'Do you take illicit drugs?'
'Who do you live with?' 'What sort of housing?' 'Are you working at the moment?'

Attempted Suicide

Scenario 2

A 20-year-old woman, Susan, has just been admitted to A&E having taken an overdose of antidepressants. Take a history and assess her suicide risk.

Introduction

'Hi Susan. My name is Jane and I'm an A&E doctor. I've been told briefly about the events this morning. I know you are probably not feeling great right now but I need to ask you a few more questions. Will that be all right?'

Assess the facts

'What happened?'
'How many tablets did you take?'
'What type of tablets were they? Did you take them with alcohol?'
'How were you discovered? Did you call the ambulance?'

Assess motive

'Why did you do it?'
'Did you intend to kill yourself?'
'Have you been planning it for a long time or was it a spur-of-the-moment decision?'
'What did you do beforehand? (write a note or a will, sort out financial affairs?)'
'Did you try to avoid being discovered?'

Past psychiatric history

'Have you tried harming yourself before?'
'Have you thought of harming other people?'

'Have you sought help from a psychiatrist/GP about your problems?'
'Are you on any medication? Are you taking it?'
'Do you think you will do it again?'

You need to elicit the underlying psychiatric problem. Is it depression (I want to die because I see no future)? Is it schizophrenia (the voice in my head said I'm no good to the world)?

Drug, alcohol and social history

'If you don't mind my asking, do you drink any alcohol?'
'Do you ever take any illicit drugs?'
'Who is at home with you?' 'Are you working at the moment?' 'Who's looking after your baby right now?'

Schizophrenia

Scenario 3

Jim, a 30-year-old man, was brought into A&E by the police. His neighbours reported some recent abnormal behaviour and alerted the police. Take a history to assess the situation.

Introduction

'Hello, Jim. My name is Jane Smith and I'm one of the doctors here. Can you tell me what's been going on?'

Elicit delusions

The patient might offer some help by saying 'I'm Jesus Christ', etc.
'Do you think other people are trying to harm you?' 'Who?' 'What do they want to do?' (persecutory delusion)
'Do you think you have special powers?' (delusion of grandeur)
'Do you think you do not exist, that part of you is dead?' (nihilistic delusion)
'Do you really think that is true?' How do you know that?' (vital questions to establish a firm belief by the patient)

Elicit hallucinations

'Are you hearing or seeing things that other people can't see or hear?'

'Do you think the voice/images are real?' (vital question to differentiate a
  hallucination from an illusion, in which the patient has the insight that the
  voices or images are false)
'Where do you think the voice is coming from?'
'How many voices are there?'
'Do they talk to you directly?' (second-person auditory hallucination)
'Do they comment on the things that you do?' (running commentary) (third-
  person auditory hallucination)
'What are they saying?'
'Do these voices describe your thoughts out loud?' (thought broadcasting)

Assess mood and past psychiatric history

'How are you feeling right now?'
'How would you describe your mood?'
'Have you previously felt very depressed or very high and excited?'
'Have you been in hospital before?' 'Is it because you were hearing the
  voices?' 'When was the last time you were in?'
'Are you on any tablets for that?' 'Do you take them regularly?'

Alcohol and drug history

Vital to exclude a drug- or alcohol-induced hallucination.

Mania

Scenario 4

Chris, a 40-year-old man, has been brought into A&E by the police. He has
been disorderly, attempted to start a fight in town, and now claims to be God
and says he is here to save the world.

Introduction

'Hello Chris, my name is Jane and I'm one of the A&E doctors. I can see that
you are very excited/very irritated. Can you tell me what's been going on?'

Establish manic behaviour

'What have you been doing in the last 24 hours?' 'What were you doing in
  town before the policemen brought you in?'

'Do you feel tired?' (excessive energy)
'Do you feel hungry?' 'Have you been eating?' (voracious appetite, or the patient might actually forget to eat)
'Have you been spending a lot of money? Where did you get your money?'
'Do you notice yourself having a higher sex drive?'
'Have you been drinking alcohol?'
'Have you taken any illicit drugs?'

Assess mood, delusions, hallucinations and past psychiatric history

'How are you feeling right now?'
'How long have you been feeling so happy and well?'
'Are you special? Do you have special talents?'
'Have you felt low and depressed before?' (Is this the manic episode of a bipolar disorder?)
'Are you seeing or hearing things that other people can't hear or see?' (Second-person auditory hallucination can occur with mania.)
'What is the voice saying?'

Anorexia Nervosa

Scenario 5

Sarah, a 16-year-old schoolgirl, was brought to your GP practice by her mother who is concerned that she has been dieting and lost too much weight. Take a history.

Introduction

'Hi Sarah, I'm Dr Smith. I understand your Mum is very concerned about your weight loss and your health. Can I ask you some questions about that?'
'First of all, do you agree that you might have lost a lot of weight?'

Assess eating habits

'How many meals do you eat a day?'
'What do you normally eat?'
'Are there certain types of food you avoid?'
'Do you eat on your own or with the rest of the family?'
'Do you binge eat?' 'Do you make yourself vomit afterwards?' (bulimia)

Elicit obsession with weight loss

'Are you happy with your weight?'
'What is your ideal weight?'
'Has anybody said you are overweight/underweight?'
'Do you weigh yourself often?'
'Does your weight change much?'
'What have you tried in order to lose weight – diet, lots of exercise, laxatives, diuretics, smoking?'

Elicit physical effects of anorexia/bulimia

'Sometimes a significant amount of weight loss can cause changes to our bodies. Have you noticed hair loss, are you still getting regular periods (amenorrhoea), have you noticed any swellings in your face (parotid glands) or changes to your teeth (erosions)?'

Precipitating factors and past psychiatric history

'Is there anything in particular that bothers you?' 'Are there any problems at school?' 'At home?'
'How would you describe your mood?'
'Have you felt depressed before?'
'Have you spoken to your friends/family/teachers about this?'

Alcohol dependence

Scenario 6

Ian is a 50-year-old man who has come to your GP practice for a sick note. He smells of alcohol, appears dishevelled and is rather irritable. Take a history.

Introduction and broaching the subject

'Good morning, Ian. I'm Dr Smith. What can I do to help?'
'I notice that you have been off sick many times lately…'
'Do you mind if I ask you a few questions about your general health and lifestyle?'
'I notice that you are a bit irritable today…'
'Have you been drinking today?'

Assess intake and drinking habits

Try to avoid interrogating or lecturing the patient, but you do need to elicit the following facts:

'How much do you drink a day?' (how many pints, glasses, bottles?)
'Is that all you drink?' 'Do you sometimes drink more than that?' (Most patients underreport initially so you need to explore further.)
'What sort of alcohol do you drink?'
'Do you also drink beer/cider/wine/spirits?'
'What time of the day do you start drinking?' 'What time do you stop?'
'Where do you go for your drinks?' (at home, pub)
'Do you drink on your own?'

Assess physical effects of alcohol

'How do you feel after a drink?'
'Are you eating well?'
'Do you suffer from stomach pains?' 'Have you ever vomited blood?' 'Have you ever blacked out?'

Assess social effects of alcohol

'How is work?'
'Where do you get the money for the alcohol?'
'Are your family/friends aware of the situation?'
'How is your relationship with your wife/parents/children?'

Assess insight and CAGE

'Do you think you have a drink problem?' (This is best preceded with CAGE questions – see page 57)

Mood, precipitating factors and psychiatric history

'Why do you think you drink so much?' 'Is there something bothering you?'
'How are you feeling in yourself?' 'How would you describe your mood?'
'Do you see or hear things that other people can't hear or see?'
'Have you seen a doctor about this before?'
'Would you be interested in any help or support with this problem?'

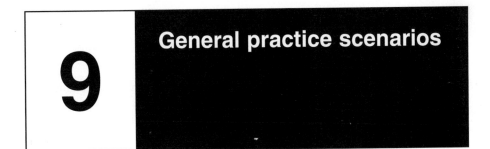

9 General practice scenarios

There are now many house officer posts which include time in General Practice. This is often reflected in final year OSCEs. It is important to remember that the setting is Primary Care rather than hospital, and that counselling and communication skills are very important. However, do not forget to deal with the presenting complaint!

Blood pressure

Scenario 1

The practice nurse has asked you to see Miss Kate Edmunds as her blood pressure has been 170/110 on two visits a month apart. Advise her.

Remember the basics

Talk to the patient and establish the reason for the interview.
Establish cardiovascular and lifestyle risk factors, previous treatment, etc.
Offer to recheck the blood pressure.
Advise her about her risk.
Negotiate lifestyle changes, investigations and treatment. Give the patient options.
Arrange follow-up and close interview.

High blood pressure

- Systolic: over 140 mmHg
- Diastolic: over 90 mmHg

Do not diagnose hypertension on the basis of one high reading! Remember that many things, including the presence of a doctor, can elevate a person's blood pressure.

Risk factors for hypertension

- Age, family history
- Diet, especially salt intake
- Sedentary lifestyle, obesity
- Smoking, alcohol, stress
- Medications
- Pregnancy
- Renal disease
- Aortic malformation
- Endocrine disorder

Medications implicated in hypertension (see page 69): steroids, alcohol, NSAIDS, the oral contraceptive pill,* antidepressants (monoamine oxidase inhibitors), as well as cocaine, amphetamine and tenamphetamine (which can cause a dangerous blood pressure rise).

At least 95% of cases are essential hypertension (no identified cause). Environmental factors are still important and occasionally a cause, and thence a cure, may be found.

Hypertension is rare in young people, especially children.

High blood pressure in pregnancy may raise suspicion of pre-eclampsia. The urine should be dipped for protein (another marker). In this case a *rise* in blood pressure is more significant than high blood pressure itself.

Remember: hypertension rarely causes symptoms.

Variables to take into account: age, sex, blood pressure, cholesterol, smoking history, diabetes mellitus, family history, ethnic origin, presence of left ventricular hypertrophy on ECG, previous cardiovascular history (see page 37).

Assessing the severity of the hypertension involves looking for signs of target organ damage:

---

*This rise in blood pressure is often mild and reversed when the oral contraceptive is stopped. Hormone replacement therapy rarely causes a rise in blood pressure.

- Ophthalmoscopy: looking for atherosclerotic changes, 'silver wiring', arteriovenous 'nipping'. In the context of a headache, retinal haemorrhages indicate malignant hypertension.
- An ECG may show ventricular strain, which may in turn suggest referral for an echocardiogram to query left ventricular hypertrophy.
- A chest x-ray may show the size of the heart or pulmonary oedema.

Tell the patient, 'Having a high blood pressure greatly increases the risk of disability or death through heart attack or stroke. However, this risk can be dramatically reduced by effective treatment'.

Treatment of hypertension

People with mild hypertension can be offered lifestyle advice initially. Therapy is indicated when the patient:

- is hypertensive despite a 'blameless' lifestyle or despite complying with lifestyle advice
- is unlikely to comply (e.g. severe arthritis, significant obesity)
- shows evidence of end-organ damage
- has a very high blood pressure (systolic >160, diastolic >100).

Scenario 2

Leroy Jones, a 60-year-old Afro-Caribbean man being treated with diuretics for hypertension, has been sent to see you by the practice nurse because after three weeks on 2.5 mg bendrofluazide daily, his blood pressure is still 170/100. Ask appropriate questions and provide appropriate advice.

An informed and agreeable patient is more likely to 'concord' with treatment. This includes warning the patient about side-effects of medications. Drug treatment is likely to be for life. However, *do not forget the basics* (above).

*Examples of (oral) drug treatments**

- **Diuretics (D),** e.g. bendrofluazide 2.5 mg each morning. *Possible side-effects:* hypokalaemia, hyponatraemia, postural hypotension, impotence.
- **β-blockers (B),** e.g. atenolol 50 mg each morning. *Possible side-effects:*

*From the *Oxford Handbook of Clinical Medicine*, Longmore M, Wilkinson I, Rajaqopalan S (eds), Oxford University Press, 2004, page 142.

bronchospasm, heart failure, cold peripheries, lethargy, impotence. *Contraindicated* in asthma and caution in established heart failure.

- **ACE inhibitors (A),** e.g. perindopril 2–8 mg each morning (may be first choice in coexisting left ventricular failure). *Possible side-effects:* cough, hyperkalaemia, renal failure, angio-oedema. *Contraindicated* in renal artery stenosis and aortic stenosis.
- **Calcium channel antagonists (C),** e.g. nifedipine MR 30–60 mg each morning. *Possible side-effects:* flushing, fatigue, gum hyperplasia, ankle oedema.

These classes of drugs can be remembered as **ABCD** (see above). When used alone, A and B are more effective in younger, white patients, B and C are more effective in older and black patients. When used in combination, A or B is added to C or D. Patients should be warned and reassured about possible side-effects, and that medication may take 4–8 weeks to take effect.

Diabetes mellitus

Scenario 3

You are the PRHO in General Practice. You have been asked to see Fred Ellis, a 20-year-old shop assistant, who presents with tiredness, weight loss and an insatiable thirst. He is terrified that he has cancer. Advise him.

What makes you suspect diabetes from a history?

A combination of any of thirst, polyuria, weight loss, unexplained tiredness, neuropathic-type numbness/pain/paraesthesia or marked visual acuity changes, as well as recurrent urinary or skin infections.

Risk factors are:

- \>65 years old
- Asian or Afro-Caribbean descent
- family history of diabetes or cardiovascular disease
- obesity, especially abdominal
- women if they have had gestational diabetes, delivery of a large baby or unexplained miscarriages (bearing in mind that pregnant women are screened for diabetes).

Diabetes mellitus (DM) is defined (WHO criteria) as a fasting venous blood glucose of over 6.7 mmol/l or a random venous blood glucose level of over 10 mmol/l (once again, this is based on more than one test several weeks apart). If the fasting value is 5.0–6.6 mmol/l or the random value is 6.7–9.9 mmol/l then an oral glucose tolerance test is indicated.

Scenario 4

You are the PRHO in General Practice. The practice nurse asks you to see Fatima LeSalle, a 67-year-old lady who is taking metformin 500 mg twice daily. This does not seem to be controlling her blood sugars; random sugars are 20 mmol/l. Furthermore, she is complaining of not being able to see as well as she used to when she drives at night. Advise her.

This station is as much about non-judgmental information gathering as it is about advice. Is she taking her medications, and what might be preventing her from complying with medications or an appropriate diet? It is worth asking questions about how she feels in herself, and then providing some counselling about her future health, perhaps negotiating a chat with the practice nurse, dietician, chiropodist and anyone else who can provide further support. Offer options rather than dictating to the patient what support they will use.

Critically, a diabetic patient who complains of loss of visual acuity must be asked if they drive. They may need to inform the DVLA (see Chapter 3). This lady should see an optician before she gets back in her car.

Complications of diabetes

- Coronary, peripheral and cerebrovascular disease
- Neuropathy
- Nephropathy
- An increased risk of cellulitis, gangrene and possible limb amputation
- Consequent renal failure, high blood pressure, foot ulcers

Scenario 5

Mrs Shelly Milligan is a heavily pregnant 34-year-old who has been referred to you as she has had glucose detected on urine dipstick on two visits to the practice, and now an oral glucose tolerance test confirms a new diagnosis of diabetes. She is alarmed at the thought of insulin injections and the possible effect on her fetus. Advise her.

Remember that you must elicit her ideas, concerns and expectations first.
Maternal diabetes is associated with:*

- polyhydramnios
- preterm labour
- stillbirth near term
- fetal macrosomia or growth restriction
- 3–4-fold increase in fetal malformations
- neonatal hypoglycaemia
- neonatal hypocalcaemia
- neonatal respiratory distress
- neonatal jaundice.

The aim is to advise the patient, without scaring her, that non-treatment is potentially more harmful than treatment with insulin.

Advice: 'Insulin is a chemical that is normally produced by the body'. However, it is not made from human cadavers and synthetic insulin has replaced bovine or porcine insulin, should this be an issue.

Whereas oral hypoglycaemics cross the placenta and may be unsafe (should the patient confess to being needle phobic), the benefits of insulin to mother and fetus clearly outweigh any risk of maternal hypoglycaemia. She should not breastfeed on oral hypoglycaemics either.

Liaison between obstetrician and diabetologist is advisable. The patient will have early scans and may need to be admitted to hospital if her blood sugars are not well controlled with subcutaneous insulin. Gestational diabetes does not always persist and she may be able to stop insulin if her oral glucose tolerance test is normal six weeks post partum. In the case of a non-insulin dependent diabetic, you would want to change them over to insulin (preconception if possible). Preconception counselling should be made available to any diabetic woman who is considering pregnancy.

Asthma

Scenario 6

Tom Williams is a 30-year-old builder who has come to your practice for the first time. He has had a persistent nocturnal cough and wheeze. He remembers being very wheezy as a child. He recently bought his daughter a puppy and wonders if he is 'allergic' to it. Advise him.

Oxford Handbook of Clinical Specialties, Oxford University Press, 2003, pages 156–7.

Suspect asthma in anyone with a chronic recurrent cough or wheeze. It can be diagnosed with two episodes of cough or wheeze which respond symptomatically to bronchodilators.

Ask about:

- symptoms: their duration and current treatment, their effect on lifestyle such as sleep disturbance, time off work, exercise intolerance
- Precipitants e.g. animals, smoke, dust, cold air, etc.
- family history
- atopy
- active and passive smoking
- occupational factors
- drugs.

This is generally a history station but state that you would:

- examine the chest
- measure the peak expiratory flow rate and compare it with the predicted value.

Management

- Discuss precipitating factors and which should be avoided (cigarettes, dust and any known allergens, possibly NSAIDs and β-blockers) and which should not be avoided (exercise) and may be helped by medication.
- It will often be sensible to prescribe a peak flow meter and teach the patient how to use it and record the values in a peak flow diary. This can be used to assess whether there is diurnal variation in PEFR or a 15% or greater improvement over two weeks/15 minutes after use of bronchodilators.
- Discuss the principles of treatment such as the use of relievers (salbutamol) and preventers such as beclomethasone.
- Teach inhaler technique, if needed, and assess inhaler technique on any poorly controlled asthmatic.
- Make an appointment for the patient to be reviewed by yourself/the practice nurse/in the asthma clinic.
- Refer to a chest physician if asthma remains poorly controlled in the long term, it is thought to be related to occupation or if the diagnosis is in doubt.

Steps in asthma management

Step 1. Occasional symptoms. Prescribe a bronchodilator as a reliever, such as salbutamol 200 μg as needed.

Step 2. If reliever is needed more than once a day, regular inhaled steroid such as beclomethasone 100–400 μg (preventer) can be given along with the PRN reliever.

Step 3. Consider increasing the dose of inhaled steroid and adding sodium cromoglycate.

Step 4. Worsening symptoms/increased need for relief. Consider long-acting β-agonists or tablets, theophyllines, inhaled tiotropium/ipratropium, high-dose (nebulized) bronchodilators.

Step 5. If control is lost, consider a short course of oral prednisolone: 40 mg for five days then 20 mg for five days.

Remember, a chronic chough and/or wheeze may be caused by lung cancer as well as other respiratory and cardiac causes. Always ask about weight loss, night sweats, haemoptysis, smoking and asbestos exposure.

Always introduce yourself as one of the doctors and establish why the medication is being given, such as steroids for COPD or warfarin for atrial fibrillation or a DVT. Ideas, concerns and expectations are very important. What does a patient know already?

Steroids

Scenario 1

David Martin is a 29-year-old journalist who has just been discharged from hospital having had an Addisonian crisis. He will need to take prednisolone and fludrocortisone for the foreseeable future. Advise him.

- Check the dose and the indication; explain why the drug is needed.
- Counsel about side-effects with high-dose/long-term steroids such as: stomach ulcers, decreased immunity, osteoporosis, weight gain and an increased risk of developing diabetes.
- 'The steroids are prescribed to…' Make sure the patient understands the benefits as well as the risks.
- 'Because we give you steroids, your body may stop producing natural steroids at times of illness, injury or increased physical stress. If you are ill or injured you should see a doctor about increasing your daily dose of steroid. This includes operations.'
- 'We will give you a steroid card in case you are ever taken ill before you are

able to get help or if you have an accident. You should carry this on you at all times.'
- A Medicalert bracelet or tag of some kind is a good idea.
- 'It is very important that you don't miss a dose, as this may make you ill, and you should let your GP know if you are stopping the steroids. This must always be done slowly if you have taken significant doses for more than a week.'
- 'We will give you an information leaflet. If you have any questions do not hesitate to contact us.'

Warfarin

Scenario 2

Mrs Charmaine Dingle is a 30-year-old woman who had a DVT and PE on returning from Australia. She recently stopped taking the combined oral contraceptive pill, as she and her husband would like to start a family. You are the PRHO and are asked to counsel her about taking warfarin.

Establish the reason for anticoagulation or confirm it. Usual examples are: AF, DVT/PE/other thrombotic/embolic events, thrombophilia, immobility and replacement heart valves.

The patient may have been on IV or subcutaneous (SC) heparin or a low molecular weight heparin SC in hospital, so you may need to explain that 'This is a tablet that you can take home with you'.

Contraindications to warfarin include peptic ulcer disease, bleeding disorders, active GI bleeding, liver failure, severe hypertension, cerebral aneurysms, endocarditis and pregnancy.

There are some side-effects. Bleeding is an obvious complication (see below) and rashes may also occur. Warfarin is *highly teratogenic* in the first trimester of pregnancy.

If a female patient plans to get pregnant, she should seek advice from an obstetrican and use contraception if sexually active in the meantime. Warfarin interferes with the oral contraceptive pill, and barrier methods of contraception should be used by women on warfarin.

The patient should also beware of interactions with other medications; the effect of warfarin is increased by **alcohol**, **aspirin**, amiodarone and chloramphenicol (and many other medications) and decreased by the **oral contraceptive pill**.

- Counsel the patient to avoid alcohol.
- The patient should tell their doctor/dentist/pharmacist that they are taking warfarin.
- A warfarin bracelet is a good idea.
- If for any reason the patient has bleeding that will not stop, they need to seek medical help from the GP or A&E. Anticoagulation with warfarin can be reversed using vitamin K or, if very severe/necessary, with fresh frozen plasma.
- If they have any questions, then they should get in touch with their doctor or the anticoagulation clinic.

'We will start by giving you a set dose and then doing a blood test.' The effectiveness of warfarin is measured using the INR. Monitoring goes from every third day to weekly to every three months* and this is done in an anticoagulant clinic or by a district nurse if a patient is immobile. The dose the patient should take will be recorded with their blood test results in a small yellow book, which also contains information about anticoagulation, and which the patient should be encouraged to read.

Anticonvulsants

Scenario 3

Mrs Jane Matthews is a 28-year-old teacher who has epilepsy and has been fit free on sodium valproate for three years. She has just started to drive again and has come into your GP practice to discuss her and her husband's desire to start a family. Advise her.

Establish why the patient is on anticonvulsants, what drug(s) they are taking and how long they have been on them.

'Have you had any problems taking the medication?' Enquire about concordance and side-effects.

Commonly used drugs and their possible toxic/side-effects[†]

- Carbamazepine: rash, nausea, diplopia, dizziness, fluid retention, hyponatraemia and blood dyscrasias.

Oxford Handbook of Clinical Medicine, Oxford University Press, 2004, pages 648–9.
[†]*Oxford Handbook of Clinical Medicine*, Oxford University Press, 2004, pages 162, 380–1.

- Sodium valproate: tremor, sedation, weight gain, hair thinning, ankle swelling, encephalopathy, liver failure.
- Phenytoin (no longer first-line therapy owing to its toxicity): decreased intellect, depression, apathy, polyneuropathy, acne, coarsening of facial features, gum hypertrophy and blood dyscrasias. Because of its toxicity this drug requires careful monitoring; ataxia, diplopia and tremor are seen in toxicity.

Most patients are seizure free within a few years of starting medication and over 60% remain so when medications are withdrawn. Risks and benefits of the medication and of perhaps stopping the medication need to be discussed. These include the patient's occupation, support, need to drive or desire to become pregnant. If medication is to be withdrawn it is usually reduced by 10% over 2–4 weeks (4–8 weeks with barbiturates). If the side-effects are not tolerated or the fits not controlled, then a different medication can be tried. The new drug is started as the old one is slowly withdrawn.

The DVLA requires that to drive, a patient must be fit free for a year and not have nocturnal fits for a year (unless there are no concurrent fits when awake and no other fits have occurred in three years).

If a patient with epilepsy wishes to become pregnant then she needs access to formal preconception counselling. Sleep deprivation and poor compliance with treatment can increase the seizure rate in pregnancy.

Epilepsy carries an increased risk* of:

- third trimester bleeding
- convulsions during labour
- prematurity, stillbirth, neonatal and perinatal death.

This is balanced against a risk of fetal malformation and developmental delay with medication, which is more common with two or more medications being taken. The risks are minimized by:

- giving the smallest number of medications needed to control the fits
- giving the lowest dose necessary to control fits
- folic acid supplements daily from preconception
- vitamin K daily from 36 weeks if taking phenytoin, primidone or phenobarbitone. The baby needs to have vitamin K at birth.
- delivering the baby in hospital because of the risk of maternal fits.

Mother and baby are reviewed postnatally. Mothers can breastfeed except with phenobarbital, which causes drowsiness in the baby. Newborns may have barbiturate withdrawal.

*Oxford Handbook of Clinical Specialties, Oxford University Press, 2004, page 161.

Part 4

Examination
skills

General guidance for physical examination stations

Know your routine

It is important to standardize your own routine for each examination. Write it down, step by step, and keep practising until you are fluent with it.

Standard examination technique

For all physical examinations, always introduce yourself and obtain consent to examine. Stand back and be seen to inspect the patient in general. Do not forget to expose the patient adequately and position them appropriately, whilst maintaining their dignity.

Practise, practise, practise

This is so important. How much you practise your routine and therefore how slick and confident you look has a direct influence on passing the exam. Those who appear unfamiliar with their work generally cannot convince the examiner that they possess 'minimum competence' and they are the ones who fail.

To talk or not to talk?

Should you describe your findings during the examination or present them at the end? The first option allows you to score points throughout the examination and is therefore strategically superior. If the examiner prefers the second option, they will probably interrupt you and ask you to present later.

Communicate with the patient throughout

You are not expected to hold a conversation during the examination but do not treat the patient like a piece of meat – interact with them! Explain what you are about to do, ask if what you are doing causes discomfort. Always enquire about tenderness before touching the patient.

Introduction

Expose and position

'I would like to expose the patient from nipples to knees, but for the sake of their dignity, I will expose just the abdomen.' Lie the patient flat, ensure he is comfortable.

General inspection

- Stand back and observe the entire patient.
- Comment on obvious findings: scars, jaundice, distended abdomen.

Hands

- Clubbing of the nails: inflammatory bowel disease (especially Crohn's disease), cirrhosis, coeliac disease.
- Signs of chronic liver disease: (leuconychia, palmar erythema, Dupuytren's contracture).
- Liver flap: a sign that liver failure has resulted in encephalopathy. Ask the patient to stretch his arms and extend his wrists. Say you would observe for 30 seconds, and move on.
- Koilonychia: iron deficiency.
- Radial pulse: rate, rhythm.
- Arteriovenous fistula (dialysis patients).

'I would normally measure the *blood pressure* now; would you like me to do so?'

Head, neck and chest

- Eyes: jaundice, anaemia
- Tongue: foetor hepaticus (liver failure); smooth (iron deficiency, β_{12} or folate deficiency)
- Neck: Virchow's node (behind left sternoclavicular joint, abdominal neoplasm spreads via thoracic duct)
- Chest: spider naevi portacath (blanch on pressing), gynaecomastia (chronic liver disease), central line, scars

Inspect abdomen

- Asymmetry
- Movement on respiration
- Pulsation
- Distension (5 Fs – flatus, faeces, fetus, fat, fluid (ascites, ovarian cyst))
- Scars (Figure 11.1)
- Caput medusae (portal venous hypertension)
- Cough (rigidity, herniae, divarification of rectus abdominis)

Palpate

'Is there any *pain* or *tenderness*?' Start away from the tender areas. Proceed to palpate at the patient's level and look at the patient's face as you palpate. Do this over each of the 9 regions of the abdomen lightly and then deeply.

- Inguinal lymph nodes: large in reticulosis or myeloproliferative disease
- Liver: start from the right iliac fossa and advance in intervals of 2 cm towards the right costal margin. Ask the patient to take deep breaths and palpate deeply on inspiration.
- Spleen: start from the right iliac fossa and advance to the left hypochondrium; five characteristics (1. site; 2. shape – notch; 3. cannot get above it; 4. moves on respiration; 5. dull to percussion)
- Kidneys: (ballot these bimanually) tender in infection, large (tumour, polycystic kidney disease, hydronephrosis)
- Masses: see Chapter 23. Consider: gastric neoplasm, omental secondaries, enlarged bladder
- Aorta: (abdominal aortic aneurysm) place your palms along the vertical midline to feel for an expansile pulsation.

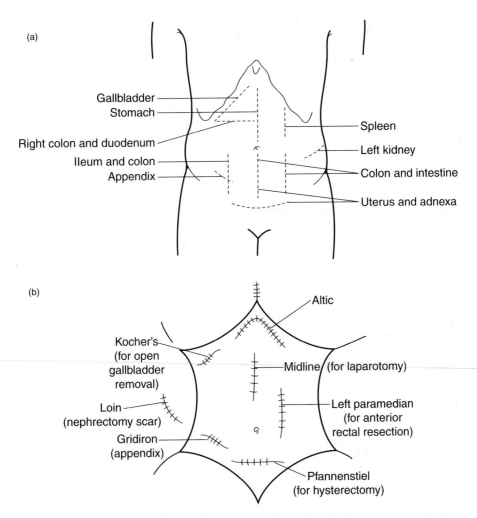

(a)

Gallbladder
Stomach
Right colon and duodenum
Ileum and colon
Appendix

Spleen
Left kidney
Colon and intestine
Uterus and adnexa

(b)

Altic
Kocher's
(for open
gallbladder
removal)
Midline (for laparotomy)
Loin
(nephrectomy scar)
Gridiron
(appendix)
Left paramedian
(for anterior
rectal resection)
Pfannenstiel
(for hysterectomy)

FIGURE 11.1 (a) Scar identification. (b) Abdominal incisions and their names.

Percussion

- Liver span: lower liver edge: percuss for dullness from the right iliac fossa to the costal margin along the midclavicular line
  Upper liver edge: percuss downwards from the 8th intercostal space. The normal liver span is ~ 12.5 cm
- Shifting dullness in ascites: percuss from the midline towards the left flank until you meet dullness. Note that spot. Roll the patient toward you and percuss that spot again. The dullness has disappeared as the fluid has shifted

- Fluid thrill in ascites: place the side of your hand in the midline and flick the side of the abdominal wall to feel a thrill

Auscultation

- Bowel sounds: tinkling → obstruction, absence → paralytic ileus, peritonitis
- Arterial bruits: aorta, renal, femoral

Examine for herniae

- Establish anatomical landmarks (namely the pubic tubercle and the anterior superior iliac spine. The femoral canal runs midway between these two points).
- 'Stand and cough, please.'
- Controlled over internal ring: indirect inguinal (passes on release towards external ring)
- Not controlled: direct inguinal
- Below and lateral to pubic tubercle: femoral

Feel for ankle oedema

Look and feel for pitting ankle oedema.

Conclude

'I would normally examine the *external genitalia* and perform a *digital rectal examination* now; would you like me to do so?'

Stations

Polycystic kidney disease (PKD)

- Bilateral, irregular, abdominal masses
- 30% have cysts in liver, pancreas
- Increased blood pressure
- FBC (↑Hb); U+Es(↑urea); US abdo; screen family members
- CT for berry aneurysm
- AV fistulae (with bruit)/Rutherford–Morrison scar – transplanted kidney?

Hepatomegaly

- Right heart failure: smooth, tender, large ± pulsatile (tricuspid regurgitation), raised JVP

- Infection: EBV, hepatitis, malaria
- Malignancy: mets or 1°, myeloma, leukaemia, lymphoma
- Others: sickle cell disease, other haemolytic anaemias, porphyria

NB: In early alcoholic cirrhosis, the liver is small.

Splenomegaly

- Infection: viral (EBV), bacterial (septicaemia), protozoal (malaria, schistosomiasis), parasitic (hydatid)
- Haematological: leukaemia (CLL/CML), lymphoma, myelofibrosis, polycythaemia, haemolytic anaemia
- Portal hypertension
- Metabolic: amyloid, storage diseases
- Cysts

If either liver or spleen is large, you must make a point to check ALL the lymph nodes.

Abdominal aortic aneurysm

- Check for other aneurysms: carotid, femoral, popliteal
- Suggest a full peripheral vascular examination
- ECG, echocardiogram
- Ultrasound scan of the abdomen: measure diameter and suggest management (watch and wait versus operate)

Renal mass

- Adult polycystic kidney disease (30–60 years)
- Renal cyst: exclude malignancy
- Hydronephrosis
- Pyelonephrosis
- Perinephric abscess
- Renal TB
- Renal cell carcinoma (male, >40 years)

12 Arterial examination

There are not too many stages in this examination but as a result, if you forget one you may miss out on a few marks.

The patient will have arterial obstruction (intermittent claudication or critical limb ischaemia), so read up on risk factors (smoking) and management (lifestyle, medical, surgical). Always compare the affected limb with the contrateral side.

Introduction

Start with six pertinent questions

- Do you have any pain in your legs? (At rest-critical limb ischaemia.)
- Which leg is worse?
- Where is the pain?
- How far up the leg does it go?
- How far can you walk? Before pain starts? (intermittent claudication)
- Do you smoke?

Expose and position

Ask the patient to remove his trousers, socks and shoes and lie on a couch.

Inspect

- (Pre) Gangrene: blackness, amputations, nail infections

- Ulceration: describe in terms of size, shape, bed, edge, slough, surrounding skin
- Venous ulcers: varicose veins, varicose eczema, painless, medial
- Arterial ulcers: **p**unched out, **p**ainful, **p**ressure **p**oints (fifth metatarsal, heel)
- Skin changes: staining, venous eczema, loss of hair, pallor
- Varicose veins
- Scars: groin, medial aspect of thigh

Palpate

'Is there any pain or tenderness anywhere?'

- Abdomen: abdominal aortic aneurysm (AAA)
- Pulses: femoral, popliteal, posterior tibialis (Figure 12.1), dorsalis pedis*
- Skin temperature
- Capillary refill time
- Any varicosities (on standing)

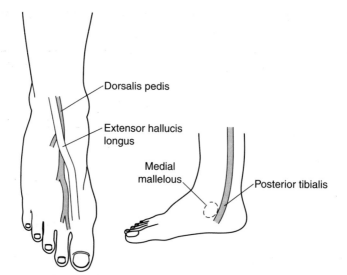

FIGURE 12.1   Pulses in the foot.

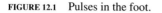

*Respectively in the groin, behind the knee, below the medial malleolus, and lateral to the first metatarsal on the dorsum of the foot.

Auscultate

'Listen for bruits. Start at the abdominal aorta. Listen to the renal and popliteal arteries.'

The aorta, common femoral arteries, superficial femoral arteries (Hunter's canal – the space located deep to the middle third of sartorius).

Buerger's test

'I would normally perform Buerger's test in both the symptomatic and asymptomatic leg; would you like me to do so?'

- Elevate leg to 45°.
- Place legs dependent at 90° over the edge of the couch (look for normal colour to return in under 10 seconds, or the presence of cyanosis and reactive hyperaemia).

Extensions

- Look at the hands and feet (to assess whether insufficiency is local or global)
- Ankle Brachial Pressure Index (ABPI)
- Duplex Doppler ultrasound, to exclude or size any suspected aneurysm
- Cardiovascular examination, Blood Pressure, CXR, AXR (calcification of the Aorta in AAA)
- Urine dipstick and BM, for diabetes (risk factor)

Remember the 6 Ps of arterial insufficiency

Pain
Pallor
Pulseless
Paraesthesia
Paralysis
Poikilothermia (perishingly cold)

Varicose veins ('examine the veins in this patient's leg')

It is unlikely that you will have a patient with 'normal' legs. There will usually be someone with varicosities and they will be obvious. Sometimes, however, patients do fail to turn up so beware a healthy person with wavy 'marker pen' lines in the distribution of a vein. Marks will be derived more from your examination technique rather than your findings.

Always remember to introduce yourself, and there is no harm in asking the patient a couple of questions such as whether they have aches in their legs, family history of varicose veins, previous DVT, problems with their blood vessels, whether anywhere is sore, etc. Also the instructions or examiner may ask you to take a two-minute history.

Examination

Ask patient to *stand* and *observe* the front and back of their legs. You are looking for:

- varicosities in the distribution of the long saphenous vein (femoral vein in groin to medial side of lower leg) and the short saphenous vein (popliteal fossa to back of calf and lateral malleolus)
- swellings
- ulcers (knowing what different types of foot ulcer looks like is an advantage)
- scars
- signs of deep venous insufficiency: haemosiderosis, venous eczema, lipodermatosclerosis.

Palpate the leg for temperature and tenderness. Look for a saphena varix (varicosity at saphenofemoral junction; thrill on cough).

To perform the *tap test*, place a finger over the saphenofemoral/saphenopopliteal junction and tap over distally placed varicosities. Valve incompetence in the veins gives rise to a thrill.

Ask patient to lie down on the examination couch. Palpate the abdomen (an abdominal mass, such as a fetus or pelvic tumour, might be putting pressure on the iliac veins), as well as the femoral and foot pulses.

Trendelenburg's test

Trendelenburg's test (Figure 12.2) detects reflux from deep into superficial veins.

Elevate the patient's legs and 'milk' (compress, moving proximally) the veins so that they no longer stand out. A tourniquet is placed around the upper thigh (occludes long saphenous vein). Stand the patient up and if:

- veins remain empty, there is saphenofemoral junction incompetence, the tourniquet has controlled it
- veins fill rapidly, there are incompetent thigh perforators below tourniquet.

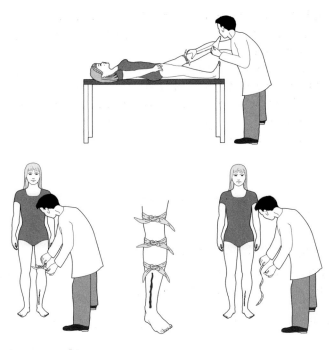

FIGURE 12.2   Trendelenburg's test.

Move the tourniquet down until the varicosities are controlled. Incompetence is **above** the level of control.

'I would normally confirm this incompetence using a *hand-held Doppler ultrasound*; would you like me to do so?' can be an excellent conclusion if you know what this involves.

Extensions

- Duplex scan
- Venography is a precursor to an operation
- Ligation or Stripping of the vein (as a form of treatment)
- Sclerotherapy (poor outcome, extremely rarely done)

13 Examination of the breast

This is not just a straightforward examination but one that requires knowledge of pathology and above all sensitivity. There are sometimes as many marks for sensitivity as there are for technique.

- Request or offer to have a **chaperone**. Elicit consent to examine.
- Sit the patient up.
- Ask eight pertinent questions (if the examiner allows).
  1. Previous lumps?
  2. Pain?
  3. Nipple discharge?
  4. Change in size related to menstrual cycle?
  5. Last period?
  6. Drugs, e.g. hormone replacement therapy, oral contraceptive?
  7. Pregnancies, details?
  8. Family history?

Expose from waist up (sit the patient at the edge of the couch)

- General inspection of patient's state of health.
- Inspection of breasts (Figure 13.1): size; symmetry; contour; colour; three signs highly predictive of cancer (nipple inversion, peau d'orange, tethering – dimpling when relaxed and/or with hands pressed on hips); axillae with hands behind head. Scars.
- Be sure to look under pendulous breasts and in the axillae.
- Ask the patient to put their hands a. by their sides b. behind their head c. on their hips, to illustrate teathering.

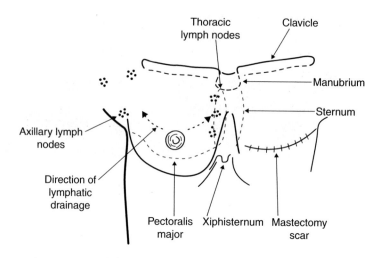

FIGURE 13.1 Anatomy around the breast including lymphatic drainage.

Sit the patient at 45°

- Examine both breasts, starting with the normal looking one.
- Ask 'Is there any *pain* or *tenderness*?' and add 'Please tell me at any point if anything is sore or uncomfortable!'
- *Palpate** all four quadrants of the breasts, across the pectoralis major and into the axillae (also examine these with arms above head).
- *Palpate* the aveolae and nipples, feeling behind the nipples for lumps. Gently compress for discharge (remember to be sensitive – you could *ask the patient to do this herself*): duct ectasia (red/green/brown), carcinoma (red) or intraductal papilloma (red). Milk from a lactating breast is a possibility. Send any discharge to cytology and microbiology.
- *Palpate lymph nodes*: expose right axillae by lifting and abducting arm by wrist with your right hand. Repeat with left regions: apical, anterior, posterior, infra/supraclavicular; medial humerus.
- Describe any nodes as you would a lump (see Chapter 23). If there is a lump, be seen to palpate the liver.
- Abdominal examination looks for evidence of liver involvement (see Chapter 11). Also look for ankle oedema.

Remember that there are points for establishing a rapport, greatly aided by the phrases 'Is there anything you are worried about? Is there anything that you would like to know?'.

*Different teachers advocate different modes of palpation. Know one, and be courteous, professional and respectful.

Extensions

- Follow up in six weeks if examination negative.
- Lumps – triple assessment:
  - clinical examination
  - aspiration and cytology; biopsy
  - imaging: <35 years of age, ultrasound; >35 years, mammography

COMMON STATIONS

Fibroadenoma

- No increased malignancy risk, resolves over years, affects women in their 30s
- Discrete, firm, mobile lump or multiple 'breast mice', not attached to skin. If it is tender or there is red discharge from the nipple, consider fibroadenosis

Fibrocystic disease

- Perimenopausal, painful swelling
- Fluctuant, smooth lump
- May be multiple, bilateral
- Slight increase in malignancy risk

Carcinoma

- Discrete lump, often hard and irregular; fixed to the chest wall
- Specialist required for staging and management. Be aware of general management – disease staging, surgery, chemotherapy, hormonal therapy, radiotherapy, breast reconstruction

Mastectomy/Lumpectomy

- What was the diagnosis?
- Are there any other scars (axillary clearance)?
- Remember to examine both the scar site and the contralateral breast.

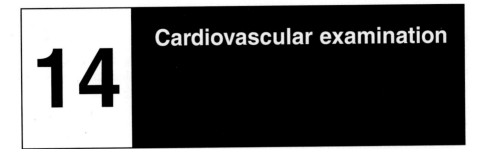

14 Cardiovascular examination

Before you begin (if permitted), ask the patient if they are experiencing any *chest pain*, *breathlessness* or *palpitations*. Have they experienced *syncope*? Although the OSCE is a contrived situation, you are subtly stating that you are on the lookout for a medical emergency.

Introduction

Expose and position the patient

Expose the chest completely, respecting the woman's dignity with a sheet or towel as necessary.

General inspection

- Breathlessness, pallor, cyanosis. Is there an oxygen cylinder in the room?
- Features of a syndrome, or congenital abnormalities (Down's or Turner's Syndromes)
- Neck Pulsation: giant a and v pulsations of JVP
- Corrigan Sign: head bobbing (aortic regurgitation)
- Listen for audible clicks of a mechanical heart valve and look for bruising (these patients are on anticoagulants)
- Scars: median sternotomy (cardiac bypass) left thoracotomy (mitral valve surgery), scars from harvesting leg veins

Hands

- Tar staining in smokers
- Splinter haemorrhages: infective endocarditis, trauma (e.g. from gardening)
- Clubbing: cyanotic congenital heart disease, infective endocarditis. Be seen to lift the hand up and observe from the side to appreciate the loss of angle between the nailbed and the finger
- CRT (capillary refill time): press on the nail bed, watch it go white and then let go. Ordinary CRT is 1–2 secs; if it is prolonged, it is abnormal and represents poor vascular supply
- Turn the hand over looking for Osler nodes, raised tender nodules on the finger pulps; or Janeway lesions, non-tender erythematous rash on the palm or finger pulps (both signs of infective endocarditis)

Radial pulse

- Rate: count the pulse over 10 seconds (looking at your watch) and give the pulse rate per minute
- Rhythm: Regular? Irregularly irregular (AF)? Regularly irregular (Wenckebach heart block)

'Do you have any pain in your shoulders? I'm going to raise your arm up'

- Collapsing pulse: lay your hand across the brachial pulse to detect this (aortic regurgitation)
- Radio-radial delay (aortic coarctation)
- Volume: ↓ – decreased cardiac output
- ↑ – CO_2 retention; thyrotoxicosis; anaemia
- State of artery: stiff in arteriosclerosis

'I would normally measure the *blood pressure* now; would you like me to do so?' This question is *mandatory* even if the answer from the examiner is usually 'no, move on'.

Eyes

Anaemia, xanthelasmata, arcus (signs of hyperlipidaemia if a young patient, may be normal in the elderly).

Tongue

Central cyanosis*

*Central cyanosis occurs where there is R→L shunting

Jugular venous pulse

Ensure the patient's head is rested against the couch and his neck is relaxed. Ask him to turn his head to the left and observe the JVP.

- Height: in centimetres above the manubriosternal angled (>3 cm is raised – right heart failure)
- Hepato-jugular reflex: if the JVP is not visible, gently press on the liver and watch it appear. Explain to the patient before doing so
- Character: these require experience to appreciate, but you need to learn the different characteristics and their causes (e.g. giant a wave – tricuspid stenosis or heartblock, large v wave – tricuspid regurgitation; see Figure 14.1)
- Kussmaul's sign: paradoxical elevation of the JVP on inspiration (constrictive pericarditis, cardiac tamponade)

The JVP has five important characteristics.

1. Complex pulsation
2. Hepatojugular reflux – $\uparrow$ 2 cm
3. Moves $\downarrow$ on inspiration
4. Cannot be palpated
5. Can be obliterated

Waveform (Figure 14.1)

a-wave – represents *atrial contraction*

- $\uparrow$ obstruction to right atrium due to RVH (right ventricular hypertrophy): pulmonary hypertension, pulmonary stenosis, tricuspid stenosis
- $\downarrow$ /absent in AF
- Cannon: closed tricuspid valve – complete heart block

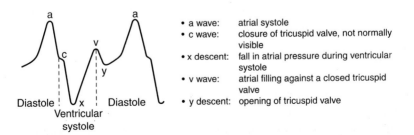

- a wave: atrial systole
- c wave: closure of tricuspid valve, not normally visible
- x descent: fall in atrial pressure during ventricular systole
- v wave: atrial filling against a closed tricuspid valve
- y descent: opening of tricuspid valve

FIGURE 14.1 The jugular venous pressure wave. *After Clinical Examination*, 4th edition, Macleod (ed.), Churchill Livingstone.

v-wave – represents *atrial filling*, closure of the tricuspid valve

- ↑ regurgitation through tricuspid in ventricular contraction: tricuspid regurgitation (TR)

y-descent – sharp in constrictive pericarditis

Carotid pulse

Palpate the carotid arteries separately.

- are they both palpable?
- bruits, listen with the bell of the stethoscope.

Palpation of the praecordium

- Apex beat: place the palm of your hand flat on the left praecordium. Define the lowest and most lateral palpable beat. **Be seen to localize it** by counting the intercostal spaces (5th intercostal space, mid-clavicular line). In cardiomegaly, the apex beat is displaced laterally.
- Heaves and thrills (palpable murmur): press your palm vertically along the right and left sternal edge

Auscultation of the praecordium

Ausculate over the four valvular areas (see Figure 14.2) for:

- Heart sounds and added sounds
- Murmurs
  - Time the murmur with the carotid pulse – is it systolic or diastolic?
  - Listen for radiation (MR → axilla, AS → carotids, AR → sternum)
  - Listen on **inspiration** to accentuate pulmonary and tricuspid murmurs, and on **expiration** to accentuate aortic and mitral murmurs
  - Posture – MS is accentuated with the patient lying on the left; AR is accentuated with the patent sitting forwards

Here is a suggested routine:

1. Listen at the apex with the bell – normal heart sounds?
2. Listen with the diaphragm and advance laterally – is there a mitral valve murmur with radiation?
3. Roll the patient to his left and listen on expiration 'Take a deep breath in, out, and then hold it.' Roll the patient back.
4. Listen in the tricuspid area and on inspiration.

5. Listen in the pulmonary area and on inspiration.
6. Sit the patient forward. Listen in the aortic area and the carotids for radiation. Listen on expiration.

Four cardiac areas (Figure 14.2)

1. Aortic area and neck – right second intercostal space
2. Pulmonary area – left second intercostal space
3. Tricuspid area – left lower sternal edge
4. Apex (mitral area) – left fifth intercostal space, mid-clavicular line

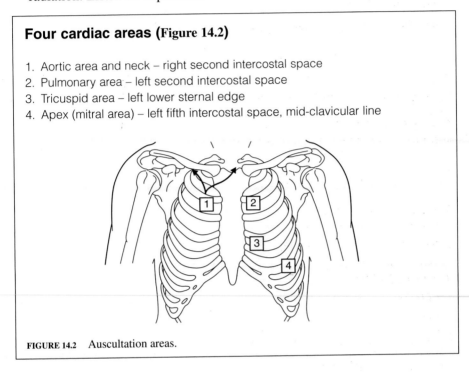

FIGURE 14.2 Auscultation areas.

Heart sounds

S_1 – sudden cessation of mitral and tricuspid flow due to valve closure
$\uparrow$ – MS; $\downarrow$ – AS, MR, LBBB; $\uparrow\downarrow$ – AF, complete heart block
S_2 – sudden cessation of aortic and pulmonary flow due to valve closure (split)
$\uparrow$ – $\uparrow$BP; $\downarrow$ – AS, PS; wide normal split – RBBB; wide fixed split – ASD

Added sounds

● S_3 – rapid ventricular filling follows S_2
S_1————-S_2-S_3
Normal in young, heart failure, constrictive pericarditis
● S_4 – atrial contraction inducing ventricular filling towards the end of diastole. Occurs with a stiff ventricle; precedes S_1:
S_4-S_1————S_2
AS, $\uparrow$BP

- Opening snap – MS after S_2
- Ejection click – AS after S_1; ↑BP
- Splitting of S_2

Auscultate of the lung bases
With the patient sitting forward
Fine crepitations in LVF

Peripheral oedema

Sacral/ankle – RVF

Peripheral pulses

Palpate liver

- Smooth, tender, enlarged – RHF
- Palpable, pulsatile and tender – TR

'To complete my examination, I would like to:'
Look at the patient's temperature chart
Examine all peripheral pulses
Examine the fundi (diabetic and hypertensive retinopathy)
Examine the abdomen for hepatomegaly
Perform urine dipstick (infective endocarditis – haematuria; hypertension – proteinuria; diabetes – glucose and proteinuria)

Murmurs*

Timing: systolic or diastolic – time against radial or carotid pulse
Site and radiation:

- MR → axilla
- AS → carotids and apex
- AR → sternum

Character:

- Pansystolic → MR, TR
- Early diastolic → AR, PR
- Mid-systolic → AS or flow murmur
- Mid-diastolic → MS

*Remember – diaphragm for high-pitched murmurs (i.e. AR), bell for low-pitched (i.e. MS).

Posture:

- MS best heard with patient lying on left (in mitral area)
- AR best heard with patient forward, holding breath after *expiration** (at the lower left sternal edge)

Respiration

- Inspiration increases murmurs of the *right* heart
- Expiration increases murmurs of the *left* heart
- Variable: pericardial rub – pericarditis

Exercise – ↑MS – no need for this in the OSCE.

Stations

Mitral stenosis

Loud S1
Opening snap
Rumbling mid diastolic murmur
Tapping apex
Best heart lying to the left on expiration

Mitral regurgitation

Pansystolic murmur
Radiates to the axilla
Thrusting displaced apex

Aortic stenosis

Plateau pulse
Systolic thrill
Ejection click
Harsh ejection systolic murmur
Radiates to carotids
Heaving apex

*It is best to demonstrate this, as most patients will take a breath and hold it. It is also kind to hold your own breath…so you know when the patient will feel uncomfortable.

Aortic regurgitation

Collapsing pulse
Soft S_2
Soft early diastolic
Murmur
Thrusting displaced apex

Tricuspid regurgitation

JVP – ↑ v-wave
No thrill
Soft pansystolic murmur, maximal at tricuspid area
Louder on inspiration
Pulsatile, tender liver

Metal prosthetic valves

May be clearly audible by the bed
Loud clicks with short flow murmur (aortic valves – systolic; mitral valves – diastolic)
Patient may have had endocarditis (clubbing) or rheumatic fever
Patient is almost certainly taking anticoagulants; extra credit may be earned if you ask them without being prompted.

FURTHER INVESTIGATIONS

Justify any investigations you recommend.

1. CXR
2. Cardiac enzymes
3. ECG
4. Exercise ECG
5. 24-h ECG tape
6. Echocardiography
7. Cardiac catheterization
8. Radioactive scan: ^{99m}Tc

15 Respiratory examination

Introduction

Exposure and position

Expose whole chest and abdomen and sit patient at 45°.

General inspection

(So … are there oxygen cylinders, inhalers, sputum pots (and their contents) lying about?).

Ask if the patient has recently experienced:

- Respiratory rate
- Breathing effort: comfortable at rest, breathless, wheezy, pursed lip breathing, use of accessory muscles
- Look around the room for sputum pot, inhaler, peak flow meter or oxygen cylinder

Hands

- Clubbing: fibrosing alveolitis, Ca bronchus, mesothelioma, bronchiectasis, lung abscess, empyema
- Peripheral cyanosis
- CO_2 retention: warm, bounding radial pulse, coarse tremor

'I would normally measure the *blood pressure* now; would you like me to do so?'

Eyes

- Anaemia
- Horner's syndrome: partial ptosis and pupil constriction (Pancoast tumour)

Tongue

Central cyanosis – COPD, severe pneumonia

Tracheal deviation

'I'm going to feel your windpipe gently, in the centre of your neck'. Palpate at sternal notch.

- Deviation away from lesion: effusion, pneumothorax
- Deviation towards lesion: fibrosis, collapse, pneumonectomy

Supraclavicular lymph nodes

TB, Ca bronchus

Inspect chest

Be seen to inspect from the front and the back.

- Scars
- Asymmetry: fibrosis, collapse
- Deformity: pectus excavatum, pectus carinatum, barrel chest (COPD – best observed from the side)

Palpation of the chest

- Apex beat: it is displaced towards the side of lobar collapse, or away from a pleural effusion.

Ask the patient to sit forward.

- Chest expansion: press your hands on the anterior chest wall, with your fingers spread and the thumbs almost meeting in the midline. Ask the patient to take a deep breath in and out, and the thumbs should part by ~5 cm. To access lower lobe expansion, squeeze the side of the chest wall until your thumbs meet and repeat the test.
- Vocal fremitus: place the edge of your hand on the upper anterior chest wall and ask the patient to say '99'. Is the vibration increased or decreased? Repeat at the corresponding location on the contralateral side for comparison. This is done at the 3 sites anteriorly and posteriorly (see area for percussion).

Percuss chest

Three clinical areas – upper, middle, lower (front and back), in order comparing left and right as you go.

- ↑ resonance: pneumothorax, emphysema
- ↓ resonance: effusion (stony dull), neoplasm
- Solid lung: consolidation, collapse, abscess (dull)

Auscultation

Listen to the breath sounds with the diaphragm of the stethoscope in the areas as you percussed. 'Take a slow deep breath in and out through your mouth'. Use the bell for the supraclavicular fossae.

- Vesicular breath sounds: louder and longer on inspiration, without a gap between inspiration and expiration (normal). See Figure 15.1
- Bronchial breath sounds: louder expiration, with a gap between inspiration and expiration (consolidation, fibrosis, pleural effusion)

Added sounds:

- Wheeze: airway narrowing
- Stridor: an inspiratory wheeze (severe airway obstruction)
- Crackles: fine (fibrosis, pulmonary oedema) or coarse (consolidation, bronchiectasis)
- Pleural rub: pleurisy (pneumonia or pulmonary infarction)

Vocal resonance

This is the auscultatory equivalent to vocal fremitus. Do either in an OSCE.

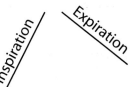

Normal

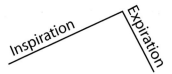

Bronchial

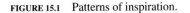

FIGURE 15.1 Patterns of inspiration.

Further investigations (these must be justified)

1. Sputum: observe and send for microscopy, culture and sensitivity or AFB*
2. O_2 saturations
3. Peak expiratory flow rate/lung function tests
4. Temperature pulse respiratory rate (charted over time)
5. Arterial blood gases
6. CXR

Potential OSCE stations

COPD

- Barrel chest
- Accessory muscles of respiration
- ↑ Resonance
- Depressed diaphragm: indrawing lower costal margin on inspiration
- ↓ Breath sounds

Asthma (acute)

- Tachypnoeic
- Expiratory wheeze
- Overinflated chest with ↑ resonance
- Pulsus paradoxus
- Enquire about allergies: commonly house dust mite or pets

Bronchiectasis

- Clubbing
- Green/yellow phlegm
- Coarse crackle over affected areas

Fibrosing alveolitis

- Clubbing
- Fine, crepitations over both bases, does not clear with coughing
- Decreased chest expansion
- Normal vocal resonance and percussion

Pleural disease

- Dry: pneumonia, infarction, cancer
- Effusion: transudate/exudate
- Stony dull to percussion

*Alcohol-acid fast bacilli – if you suspect a *Mycobacterium* infection, essentially TB.

16 Cranial nerve examination

Cranial nerve functions

Many cranial nerves have multiple functions and not all of them can be easily tested in an OSCE. Table 16.1 shows those that you are expected to test in an exam situation.

Testing reflex pathways

All reflexes have an afferent and an efferent pathway, subserved by different nerves. Be clear about the signs that indicate dysfunction in each pathway.

Pupillary reflex

- Afferent: light perception – optic nerve (II)
- Efferent: pupillary constriction – oculomotor nerve (III)

Corneal reflex

- Afferent: corneal sensation – ophthalmic division of trigeminal nerve (Vi)
- Efferent: blinking – facial nerve (VII)

Gag reflex

- Afferent: laryngeal sensation – glossopharyngeal nerve (IX)
- Efferent: gag – vagus nerve (X)

TABLE 16.1   Cranial nerve functions

Cranial nerve	Functions	What to test in an OSCE
I Olfactory	Smell	Ask about sense of smell and taste appreciation
II Optic	Visual acuity	Reading print, Snellen chart
	Colour vision	Ishihara plates, red desaturation
	Pupil construction (afferent pathway)	Pupillary reflexes
	Visual field	Confrontational field test
III Oculomotor	Lid elevation	General inspection for ptosis
	Pupil constriction (efferent pathway)	Pupillary reflexes
	Ocular motility MR, SR, IR, IO	Extraocular movement
IV Trochlear	Superior oblique	Extraocular movement
V Trigeminal	Facial sensation	Test sensation of face
	Corneal sensation	Corneal reflex
	Facial motor temporalis and masseter	Gritting teeth
VI Abducens	Abduction of eyes	Eye movement
VII Facial	Facial motor	Facial expressions
VIII Vestibulo-cochlear	Hearing	Screening of hearing Rinne's and Weber's tests
	Balance	*Not tested*
IX Glossopharyngeal	Pharyngeal sensation	Gag reflex
	Phayryngeal motor, autonomic to parotid gland	*Not tested*
X Vagus	Motor to pharynx	Gag reflex Soft Palate
	Motor to larynx, autonomic, sensory to external auditory canal	*Not tested*
XI Accessory	Sternocleidomastoid	Shoulder shrug
XII Hypoglossal	Tongue movement	Tongue protrusion

Eye examination (II, III, IV, VI)

'Please examine this patient's eyes.'

Examination of the eyes should proceed in the following order.

1. General observation
2. Visual acuity
3. Eye movements
4. Visual fields
5. Pupils
6. Fundus examination with an ophthalmoscope (if this is not expected, the examiner will stop you at this point)

Leave any tests that involve a torch till *last* as it will 'blind' the patient with a ghost shadow. Always start with visual acuity, as you need to ascertain whether the patient can see reasonably before performing tests that require the patient to follow a target (eye movements, fields).

General observation

- Ptosis: total/ partial
- Ocular deviation: IIIrd nerve palsy
- Pupillary asymmetry
- Proptosis: thyroid disease, orbital masses

Visual acuity

This is the 'clarity' of vision. Always test acuity with the patient's glasses on as they correct any refractive error. Any uncorrected visual loss can therefore be assumed to be retinal or neurological in origin. Remember to test each eye separately.

Reading print

This is a crude but simple and quick test, probably all you are expected to do in an OSCE. The examiner might provide you with a printed card or you may be expected to improvise, e.g. with your name badge, instructions card in the exam room, etc.

Glasses off

From this point onwards, all eye tests are done with the glasses off, as they act as an obstruction in visual field testing and reflect off the light you shine into the eyes.

Eye movements

There are six extraocular muscles. Some of them have multiple and overlapping actions and cause the eyes to move in more than one direction. Below is a simplified account of the movements of each muscle and their nerve supply.

- IIIrd nerve: upgaze (superior rectus), downgaze (inferior rectus), adduction (medial rectus), upgaze and adduction (inferior oblique)
- IVth nerve: downgaze and adduction (superior oblique)
- VIth nerve: abduction (lateral rectus)

Testing eye movements

- Gently steady the patient's head. Ask the patient to look straight ahead and observe the eye position.
- Put your finger out about a foot in front of the patient.
- 'Keep your head still. Follow my finger with your eyes, and tell me if you see double.'
- Move your finger in a big H to the extremes of gaze. It is normal to get a small degree of nystagmus at the extremes of gaze.

In testing eye movements, you are looking for:

- eye position on primary gaze
- full, smooth, conjugate eye movements. No nystagmus
- diplopia on eye movements.

Abnormal eye movements (Figure 16.1)

- IIIrd nerve palsy: eye assumes the down-and-out position on primary gaze. Limited movement in most directions except abduction. Associated ptosis and possibly dilated pupil as well.
- IVth nerve palsy: affected eye *cannot* look down and in.
- VIth nerve palsy: limited abduction.
- Nystagmus: causes include cerebellar disease (pendular nystagmus), vestibular disorder, physiological (on extreme gazes), congenital.
- Internuclear ophthalmoplegia: this is caused by a lesion of the medial longitudinal fasciculus. It may be damaged by demyelination (usually bilateral) or vascular disease (unilateral). This produces symptoms of horizontal diplopia and causes reduction of adduction on the side of the lesion and nystagmus of the contralateral abducting eye.

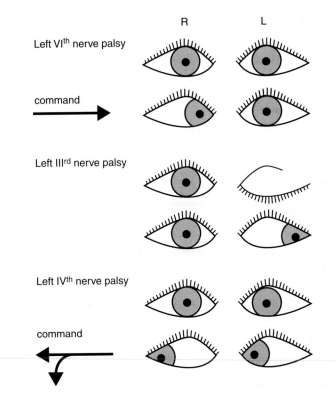

FIGURE 16.1 Abnormal eye movements for IIIrd, IVth and VIth nerve palsy of the left eye.

Pupils

Elicit the following:

- symmetry of pupils
- direct reflex
- consensual reflex
- accommodative reflex
- exclusion of relative afferent papillary defect (RAPD).

Proceed as follows:

1. Dim the room light. Instruct the patient to look far ahead at a target such as a light switch. Otherwise, fixating on a close target (accommodation) causes pupil constriction (accommodative reflex). Position yourself to the side of the patient and do not obstruct their view of the target.
2. Inspection: remember to look for pupil asymmetry, such as in IIIrd nerve palsy (ipsilateral dilated pupil) or Horner's syndrome (ipsilateral constricted pupil).

3. Shine a light from the *side* of the eye to ensure that only one eye is illuminated.
4. Observe for direct reflex in the ipsilateral eye, then shine the light again at the same eye and look for consensual reflex in the contralateral eye. Repeat with the other eye.
5. Accommodation: ask the patient to fixate at a distant target. Look at their pupils. Place a pen or finger at a close distance in front of them and ask them to look at that. You should see both pupils constrict and the eyes adduct.
6. Relative afferent papillary defect (swinging light test/ Marcus Gunn pupil). Ask the patient to fixate on a distant target. Shine the light alternately several times from one eye to the other. A paradoxical dilation of the pupil when light is shone is indicative of an RAPD on that side. RAPD is due to damage to the ipsilateral optic nerve.

Confrontational visual fields

The bedside visual field test is done by confrontation, i.e. testing the patient's fields against yours. Remember to test one eye at a time, as the two eyes' central fields intersect.

1. Sit facing the patient about one arm's length apart, adjusting the height of your seats so that you are at the same eye level.
2. Ask the patient to cover his right eye with his right hand and to keep looking at your nose. Cover your left eye with your left hand.
3. Slowly move a target from the peripheral field towards the centre. Ask him to say 'yes' the moment he can see the target. Ensure he is always fixating at your nose and you should be looking at his. Repeat for all four quadrants of the visual field and then the other eye.

It's acceptable to use your finger as the target. Sometimes a white/red hatpin is provided, which acts as a well-defined target. Our central vision is most sensitive to red and the periphery to white but it is acceptable to use the red pin for the whole exam. Ensure that the target is always midway between you and your patient.

How to assess the size of the blind spot

The blind spot corresponds to where the optic nerve enters the eye. It is enlarged in papilloedema. You can find your own blind spot by covering one eye and looking straight ahead. Hold a red hatpin out and move it horizontally. It will disappear initially and then reappear. The area across which this happens corresponds to the blind spot.

To assess the patient's blind spot against yours, sit directly opposite each other and cover one eye (your right eye against the patient's left). Hold a red hatpin out and ask him to tell you when it disappears and reappears again. The area across which this occurs will be wider than yours if the patient has an enlarged blind spot.

Visual field defects

Field defects can result from damage to any part of the visual pathway. All lesions behind the optic chiasm are homonymous (same side in each eye) and they are due to contralateral lesions.

Possible OSCE cases

- Monocular blindness: ipsilateral ocular (e.g. eye trauma, advanced cataracts) or advanced optic nerve abnormalities.
- Bitemporal hemianopia: due to compression of the optic chiasm, classically due to pituitary tumours.
- Homonymous hemianopia: contralateral optic tract or occipital lobe lesions.
- Macula-sparing homonymous hemianopia: the macula region of the retina is responsible for central vision. Its fibres project to the tip of the occipital lobe. An occipital infarct that spares the tip will therefore produce macula-sparing homonymous hemianopia, where the central area of vision is spared.

How to use an ophthalmoscope

An ophthalmoscope provides a magnified but restricted view of the fundus. Use your right eye to test the patient's right eye to avoid the embarrassing 'kissing' position.

Before you begin, check the ophthalmoscope. Turn it on, shine it on your hand and get the largest and brightest setting (the largest circular spot) by turning the dial. The set of dials with numbers adjusts the clarity of view. Set it to 0.

1. Explain what you're doing for full cooperation. 'I'm going to examine the back of your eye with this bright torch. I'll have to move very close to you (*warning*) to do so. Let me know if you're getting uncomfortable and we can stop (*show consideration*). Is that all right (*gain consent*)?'
2. Ask the patient to remove his glasses. Dim the room to obtain dilated pupils. Tell the patient to focus on a well-defined object far ahead. 'Look at the light switch on the wall and keep staring at it. Even if I get in your way.'

3. Check for the red reflex. Stand about one metre away and to the side of the patient. Shine the light into each eye and look through the ophthalmoscope to see a bright red reflex from the retina through the pupil. An absent red reflex (which looks dull and grey) or a white reflex indicates opacity in the ocular media (e.g. a cataract) or retinal abnormalities (retinal detachment, masses).

4. Examination of the fundus (Figure 16.2). Stand about a foot from the patient on the side you're testing. Look through the ophthalmoscope with your right eye to examine the patient's right eye. Move towards him until you are close enough to see retinal details (optic disc, blood vessels), which is usually very close.

If fundal details are blurred, try turning the dial; this corrects any blurring due to short- or long-sightedness in you or your patient.

Follow the vessels into the optic disc, where they converge. Try and follow the other vessels that radiate from the disc and look into the four quadrants of the peripheral retina.

Arteries are narrower and they travel on top of the veins. The macula is the area of retina temporal (lateral) to the optic disc. It is important for central vision.

Repeat for the other eye, starting by standing one foot away and moving in again.

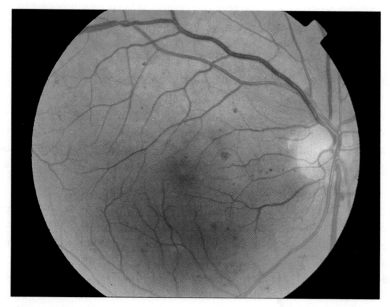

FIGURE 16.2   Fundus of the eye.

Possible signs in OSCE fundal examination

- Healthy optic disc: clear margins, yellow colour
- Blurred optic disc margin/papilloedema: the term 'papilloedema' describes a blurred disc margin specifically due to raised intracranial pressure
- Optic atrophy: pale (white) optic disc
- Diabetic retinopathy (Figure 16.3):
  - background: dot blot haemorrhages, microaneurysms, soft exudates
  - pre-proliferative: hard exudates, intraretinal microvascular abnormalities (IRMA) – shunt vessels between the retinal veins and arteries, cotton wool spots (ischaemic nerve fibres in the retina)
  - proliferative: neovascularization on the disc (NVD) or elsewhere in the retina (NVE). These can be very subtle and require experience to detect
- Hypertensive retinopathy: AV nipping, silver wiring, flame-shaped haemorrhages, exudates, cotton wool spots, blurred disc margin
- Central retinal artery occlusion: retinal pallor (instead of healthy orange colour) affecting all four quadrants, cherry-red spot
- Central retinal vein occlusion: dilated tortuous veins, widespread haemorrhages, cotton wool spots
- Branch vein/artery occlusion: as the above but only affecting the corresponding quadrant(s) of the retina, each supplied by a branch of the central retinal artery/vein

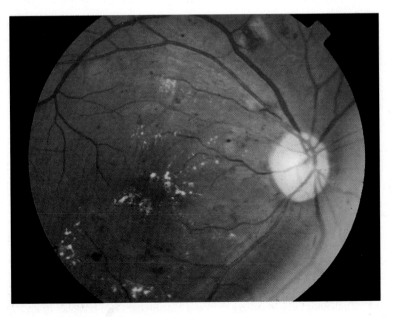

FIGURE 16.3   Diabetic retinopathy.

Examination of the face (V, VII)

Facial sensation

- Ask the patient to close his eyes.
- Test sensation by gently touching both sides of the face, at three spots corresponding to the three divisions of the trigeminal nerve (see Figure 16.4).
- Stay close to the midline as the peripheral areas of the face are supplied by the occipital nerves.
- Ask the patient if (1) he can feel both sides; (2) they feel the same.

Corneal reflex

Two nerves are being tested in the corneal reflex:

1. the ophthalmic division of the trigeminal (afferent), which supplies corneal sensation
2. the facial nerve (motor efferent), when the patient blinks.

Roll up some tissue into a thin tapered end. Ask the patient to look straight ahead and gently touch the cornea (over the coloured part of the eye) with the tissue. The patient should respond with blinking. Approach the patient from the side as many people will blink in anticipation of seeing the tissue.

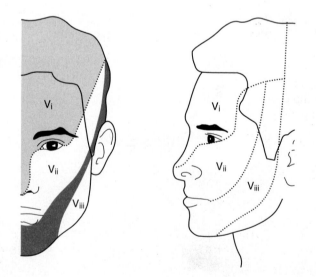

FIGURE 16.4 Opthalmic (Vi), Maxillary (Vii) and Mandibular (Viii) branches of the trigeminal nerve.

Trigeminal motor

Do not forget that the trigeminal nerve supplies two muscles in the face: temporalis and masseter. Test them straight after facial sensation to show the examiner that you know they are supplied by the trigeminal nerve.

Simply ask the patient to grit his teeth, then feel his temples and jaws for the muscle bulk. Then ask the patient to open his mouth and try to close it.

Facial motor function

Always remember to be seen to observe the face for asymmetry. It's tempting to overdo the facial motor testing as they are fun to perform but stick to a maximum of three.

1. Always test frontalis function. 'Raise your eyebrows.' This is an important test in the presence of a facial palsy, to differentiate an upper motor neurone VII lesion (sparing of function) from a lower motor neurone lesion (inability to raise eyebrow).
2. 'Close your eyes tight.' Try to prize open patient's eyelids – gently.
3. 'Blow your cheeks out.'

Examination of the ears and hearing (VIII)

Screening hearing test

Whisper a number in one ear as you mask the other with the rustling of your fingers. Ask if he can hear that. Repeat with the other ear and ask if it sounds as loud. Is it the same on both sides?

Examination of the mouth (IX, X)

- General observation
- Soft palate movement
- Gag reflex
- Tongue movements

Ask the patient to open his mouth and observe the tongue for wasting and fasciculation as it rests in the mouth.

Ask the patient to say 'ah' and observe the soft palate movement. It should move up centrally. It deviates to the contralateral side in a vagus nerve lesion.

Gag reflex

Use a tongue depressor to touch the posterior pharyngeal wall. The soft palate will lift up and the patient gags.

The gag reflex is rarely tested in an OSCE as it is uncomfortable for the patient.

Tongue movements

- Protrusion: 'Stick your tongue straight out'. The tongue will deviate towards the side of weakness (e.g. hypoglossal nerve palsy).
- Tongue power: 'Push your tongue against the inside of your cheek'. Resist the patient's tongue from the outside of the cheek.

Suggested OSCE routine for cranial nerve exam

'Please examine this patient's cranial nerves.'

Introduction

'Good morning, my name is John Smith. I'm a final-year medical student. Do you mind if I examine the nerves on your head and neck? Thank you.'

Smell

'Firstly, do you notice any changes in your sense of smell or taste?'

General inspection

Step back and take a hard look at the patient's face for facial asymmetry, ptosis, ocular deviation and pupil asymmetry.

Eyes

'I'm going to test your vision now. Can you please put your glasses on? Cover your right eye with your right hand. Read the letters on this chart/sentence on this card.'

'Now cover your left eye with your left hand and read the letters again.'

'Now I'm going to test the movement of your eyes' (*first observe the eyes for deviations, asymmetry of pupils*). 'Just keep your head still' (*gently steady patient's head*). 'Now follow my finger with your eyes and tell me if you see double.'

(*Position patient at the same level and directly facing you*). 'I'm now going to test your visual fields. I'd like you to cover your right eye with your right hand and keep looking at my nose. Say "yes" the moment you see my finger/the red pin move into the corner of your vision' (*repeat for four corners of visual field*).

'Now cover your other eye up and do the same.'

'I'm now going to shine a light into your eyes. Just keep looking straight ahead at the light switch' (*first inspect the pupils, then test direct and consensual pupillary reflexes*).

'Now keep looking at the light switch' (*look at pupils, then hold a target close to patient*). 'Now look at my pen here' (*accommodation reflex*).

Face

'I'm now going to test the feeling on your face. Close your eyes' (*gently touch division of Vi*). 'Can you feel that? Does it feel the same on both sides?' (*repeat for Vii and Viii*) 'Does this feel the same as before? Same on both sides?'

'Grit your teeth' (*feel for masseter and temporalis*). 'Raise your eyebrows. Close your eyes tightly' (*gently try to prise open eyelids*). 'You can open your eyes again.'

Hearing

'Now can you hear that?' (*rustle fingers against one ear*) 'Does it sound the same on the other side?' (*repeat with other ear*).

Mouth

'Open your mouth and say "ah"' (*look at soft palate movement*). 'Stick your tongue out' (*look for deviation*). 'Push against the inside of your cheek' (*as you push against it from outside*) 'and repeat with the other side.'

Neck and shoulders

(*Put your hands on patient's shoulders*) 'Shrug your shoulders and keep them up' (*try and push shoulders down*).

(*Put your hand against patient's cheek*) 'Now push your cheek against my hand' (*look at sternocleidomastoid then repeat for other side*).

'Thank you very much.'

'To complete my examination, I'd like to:

- test the corneal reflex
- examine the fundi with an ophthalmoscope
- test the gag reflex
- test hearing formally with a tuning fork'

(or suggest other tests relevant to the history and significant examination findings, e.g. test gait and cerebellar system if there is nystagmus; examine fundi in a diabetic.)

17 Dermatological examination

This can take one of two basic forms:

1. Take a brief history and examine the patient's skin.
2. This patient has come in to ask about something skin related. Elicit a history and/or advise them.

Always introduce yourself, establish the patient's details and establish a rapport.

Taking a dermatological history

- Presenting complaint (rashes, moles, etc.)?
- History of presenting complaint?
- Site and distribution of the skin lesion?
- Has this changed, got better or worse?
- Is it itchy, and is this localized or generalized?
- Is there any pain or disturbed sensation associated with the lesion?
- Are there any systemic symptoms (weight loss, fatigue, headache, joint pain and stiffness where relevant)?
- Any changes associated with hair and nails or at the hairline?
- Any previous treatment? 'Have you tried anything for it? Have you been to see anyone about this before?'
- Any past history of skin problems, allergies or atopy?
- Past medical history?
- Drug history? Any known drug allergies?
- Occupation, hobbies (exposure to an irritant or noxious substance)?

- History of excessive sun exposure (e.g. sunbed use, frequent sunbathing, lived in tropical countries?)
- Pets?
- Family history of skin problems (atopy, possible infestations, skin cancers)?
- Functional history: how is the patient affected by his skin condition? Does the itch disturb his sleep or work? Is he embarrassed by his appearance? What are his ideas, concerns and expectations?

The examination

Ask the patient to expose the area they are concerned about and state that you would examine as much of the skin as possible. Ask the patient if they have noticed lesions anywhere else on their body. Express a desire to examine the entire body and be seen to look at both sides of the hands, the nails and the hairline.

How to describe a skin condition

Expose – Ask the patient to expose the area they are concerned about. Ask if he has noticed any lesions elsewhere on his body. Remember to examine the hands, nail and hairline. Say you would like to examine the entire body normally.

How to describe a Skin lesion

- Distribution: is it symmetrical, peripheral or mainly on the trunk. Is there a photo-expose distribution? Is it on flexor or extensor surfaces?
- Number of lesions
- Size and shape, colour
- Surface texture (scaly/crusted/ulcerated), raised/flat
- Terminology: can the lesions be described by the following terms?

Flat lesions: Macule, patch
Raised solid lesions: papule (<1 cm), nodule (>1 cm), plaque, weal, wart
Fluid filled lesions: cyst, blister, vesicle, pustule, abscess
Broken surfaces: ulcers, fissures, erosions

Be able to recognize and talk about acne (Figure 17.1), eczema (Figure 17.2), psoriasis (Figure 17.3), keloid (Figure 17.4), contact dermatitis, pityriasis, melanoma (Figure 17.5) and basal cell carcinoma (Figure 17.6) as well as fungal skin infections. You may want to watch out for the odd rarity such as the café-au-lait patches associated with neurofibromatosis.

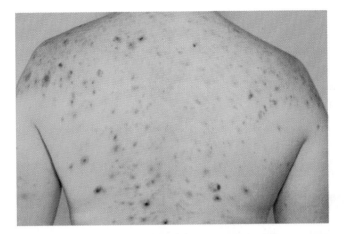

FIGURE 17.1   Acne.

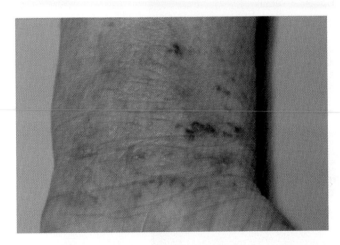

FIGURE 17.2   Eczema.

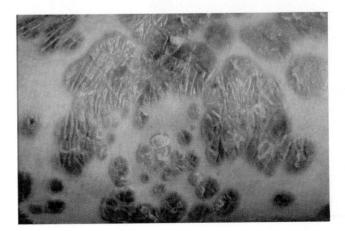

FIGURE 17.3   Psoriasis.

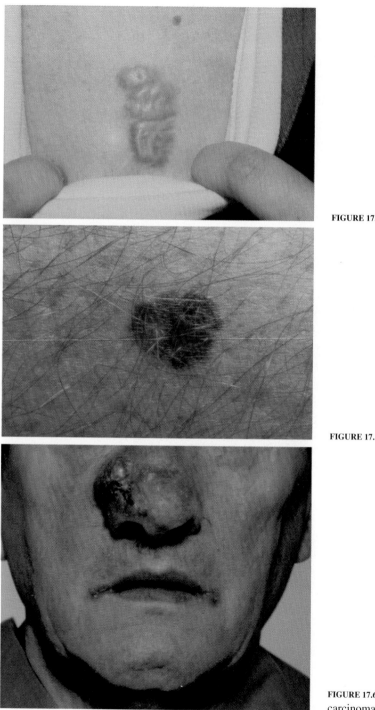

FIGURE 17.4 Keloid.

FIGURE 17.5 Melanoma.

FIGURE 17.6 Basal cell carcinoma.

It may be appropriate to suggest an investigation:

- Skin swab: microscopy, culture and sensitivity (e.g. ulcers)
- Skin biopsy if there is diagnostic doubt. Excision of the lesion if malignancy is suspected.
- Patch testing: allergies
- Skin scrapings and microscopy: fungi and parasites
- Wood's light: highlights white areas in white skin, e.g. with fungal infections

Possible OSCE stations

- **Mrs Jones is a 30-year-old lady who had a mole excised two weeks ago in clinic. The mole was in fact a melanoma less than 2 mm thick and was excised with a clear margin. No lymphadenopathy was felt at previous clinics and no satellite lesions were seen. She has come for the results of the biopsy. Advise her.**

  Establish her ideas, concerns and expectations *before* you give any new information. Tell her the bad news that it was a malignant mole *and* the good news (that the mole was completely excised, etc.). The patient will be anxious and upset with the news and you may need to hear her concerns before proceeding. Establish the risk factors. Advise her to have mole checks. Advise reduced sun exposure, ultraviolet protection creams, etc. She will need to be followed up and explain the possible need for re-excision, which is standard treatment.

- **Mrs Smith is the anxious mother of two toddlers, who has come to you for advice on what sun protection is best for them. Advise her.**

  Establish her ideas, concerns and expectations. Find out what she already knows. Establish why she is anxious, e.g. something on the television?
  Young children are advised to wear hats and appropriate clothes or sunblock during hot sunny weather in the summer.

- **You are the PRHO in General Practice. You are asked to see Jane Smith, a 16-year-old schoolgirl with increasingly severe acne. She has returned to the surgery because twice-daily washing with coal tar soap has not helped and she is increasingly unhappy with her condition.**

  Explore her ideas, concerns and expectations. Emphasise that this condition is very common in teenagers. Check her compliance to treatment. Explain that treatment often takes 3 months to result in any improvement. Reassure her that there are many other available treatments (e.g. antibiotics or the contraceptive pill). Suggest a new treatment if appropriate and reassure her that she will be seen regularly to assess her response. Agree on a plan.

- **You are the PRHO in General Practice. The Health Visitor has asked you to speak to Mrs McShane as the Health Visitor is convinced that her two-year-old daughter Dorothy has scabies.**

  You need to establish what Mrs McShane already knows, whether she has noticed the skin problem and what she thinks it is due to, before launching into the diagnosis and its treatment, which will involve checking all the family in contact with Dorothy and possibly letting a nursery know. This needs to be done in a tactful manner.

Examination of the ear

Introduction

ENT teaching is generally highly sought after by finalists. If you are reading this with some time left before finals, at the very least, it is worth finding a friendly ENT clinic, Registrar or Consultant to go through examination of the ear.

As with any examination station in an OSCE, gain consent and establish patient identity and rapport. The ear examination is usually combined with a brief history (you will be told if this is the case – *if in doubt, ask*). The *presenting complaint*, history of presenting complaint and *how it affects the patient* are vital. The rest of the history can be broken into five screening questions and five risk factors. There are closed questions to elicit key data. Marks will mostly be awarded for fluent and correct examination technique.

Screening

Is there any:

- hearing loss
- pain/itch
- discharge
- tinnitus (which ear?) 'Do you hear a ringing noise in your ear'
- vertigo? 'Does the room spin round and make you dizzy?'

Risks

- Family history
- Head trauma

- Medication (especially aminoglycosides and NSAIDs)
- High noise levels
- Previous ENT problems

Of course, you may ask about other relevant issues like whether someone with earwax and recent onset of pain and deafness has been swimming.

Examination

Explanation

'May I examine the inside of your ear with this instrument? It may be slightly uncomfortable but should not be painful. Is your ear painful to touch?

Position

Ask the patient to take a seat while you sit 90° facing the patient's ear.

Outer ear

Inspect for: hearing aid, scars, inflammation and vesicles of the pinna.
Palpate for: mastoid tenderness, pre-auricular lymph nodes.
Pull on the pinna gently – it is tender in external ear diseases.

Introduce the auroscope, and attach a clean disposable tip. Correct use of the auroscope involves holding it like a pen rather than a hammer, allowing you to steady it against the patient's face with your little finger and to gently pull backwards on the patient's pinna with the other hand (Figure 18.1). Though you may not see it all at one go, you should be able to identify the eardrum and its features and anything abnormal (Figure 18.2).

Inspection through auroscope

External Auditory Canal

- Wax
- Foreign body
- Discharge (mastoiditis, otitis externa, acute and chronic suppurative otitis media)
- Blood (bullous myringitis)
- Boils (furunculosis)

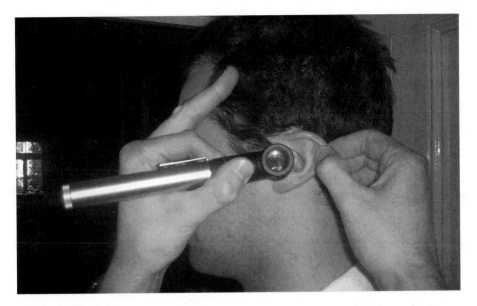

FIGURE 18.1 Correct use of the auroscope.

Tympanic membrane

- Normal pearly colour
- Boggy and inflamed (acute and chronic suppurative otitis media)
- Haematoma (trauma)
- Perforation (otitis media, trauma)
- Blisters (bullous myringitis)

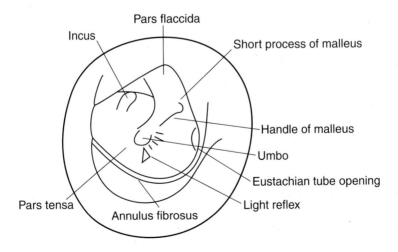

FIGURE 18.2 Diagram of the eardrum.

Bedside hearing test

Whisper a number in one ear while you either occlude the other ear by the tragus (tragel rubbing) or mask it with a noise, such as the rustling of your fingers. This test only identifies a gross hearing deficit.

Rinne and Weber's tests

The tuning fork needed for these tests is 512 Hz- the number '512' should be engraved on it. It is actually difficult to prong, so just strike it on something firm, such as your knee or elbow, but never on the patient!

Rinne test – Compare sounds heard by air and bone conduction.
Explain to the patient: 'Tell me which is louder – one or two?'

Activate the tuning fork and hold it so that both prongs are in line with the patient's ear (air). Say 'one'. Then press the base to the mastoid process (bone) – say 'two'.

- Air louder than bone: normal or sensorineural deafness
- Bone louder than air: conductive deafness

Weber's test – To lateralize the deaf ear.
Place the base of the activated tuning fork on the centre of the patient's forehead (not over his hair!) or the bridge of his nose. Ask 'Where do you hear the sound?'

- Normal hearing: centrally
- Conductive deafness: heard in the good ear
- Sensorineural deafness: heard in the deaf ear.

Naturally there are marks for summarizing the findings, identifying the pathology, thanking the patient and asking them if they have any questions. *Always* ask how their problem is affecting them.

You may wish to suggest:

- referral to an ENT surgeon (e.g. in pain/conductive deafness)
- syringing, olive oil drops (for ear wax)
- audiometry
- head CT (in sensorineural deafness)

or any other relevant referral or procedure for extra points.

19 Gait examination and GALS screening

Gait

Throughout the gait examination, ensure the patient does not fall. Help them on and off the bed, walk *alongside* them, and be heard to say 'I will catch you if you fall' to get the extra marks.

Order of tests:

- Observation
- Standing with feet together
- Standing with feet together and eyes closed (Romberg's sign)
- Walking: short walk by the bedside, heel-to-toe (tightrope) walking, heel walking.

Observation

- Does the patient have an abnormal posture?
- Stooped, with little armswing – Parkinsonism.
- Can the patient walk unaided? Do they rely on a stick or frame?

Romberg's sign

Ask the patient to stand with their two feet together. Then ask them to close their eyes and see if they are more unsteady. Positive Romberg's sign is the *increase* in unsteadiness with eyes closed compared with when the eyes are open. It is indicative of sensory ataxia.

- Sensory ataxia: loss of proprioception due to posterior column lesion in the spinal cord (e.g. cord compression due to spondylosis or tumour, vitamin B12 deficiency, tabes dorsalis). Patients rely on visual cues for balance, so unsteadiness is *worse with eyes closed.*
- Cerebellar ataxia: these patients are generally unsteady whether with eyes open or closed. Romberg's sign is *negative.*

Walking

- Bring the patient somewhere spacious to watch them walk. Walk *with* the patient in case they fall.
- Ask them to walk in a straight line, turn around, and walk back towards the starting point.
- Heel-to-toe walking can exacerbate existing unsteadiness but practise on enough 'normal' individuals and you will realize it is not always easy.
- Heel walking is tested to highlight weakness of the gastrocnemius.

What to look for

1. Is the gait steady, symmetrical and smooth?
2. Do they have any characteristic gait?
   - Shuffling gait: Parkinsonism
   - High stepping: knees lifted high to compensate for the foot drop
   - Hemiplegic gait: one leg swings out to the side. This is due to unilateral upper motor neurone lesion (i.e. a stroke)
   - Broad-based gait: the feet are wide apart as the patient is unsteady. Causes include sensory or cerebellar ataxia
   - Waddling gait: the pelvis rotates markedly, due to proximal muscle weakness
   - Antalgic gait: the patient appears in pain. They most likely appear in the rheumatological rather than the neurology exam

Parkinsonism

The three diagnostic features are:

- rest (pill rolling) tremor
- bradykinesia
- cogwheel rigidity.

Other common features include stooped posture, mask-like facies, micrographia.

GALS (gait, arms, leg, spine) screening

This is a set of quick-to-perform examinations that make ideal OSCE questions. GALS is a simple musculoskeletal screen for functional disability. Be systematic in the examination and presentation of findings.

Introduction

Exposure

Ask the patient to remove their top and trousers to expose their arms, legs, neck and back.

Screening questions

'Do you suffer from any pain or stiffness in your arm/leg, back/neck?'
'Do you have any difficulty with washing and dressing or with steps and
  stairs?'

Gait

Observe posture.
Ask patient to walk and watch for a normal symmetrical gait.
Ask the patient to sit down and then get up from a chair.

Arms

Sit the patient down and ask them to show you their hands.
Observe both surfaces for swellings and deformities.
Demonstrate the following and ask the patient to copy you:

- power grip (see Figure 20.3)
- precision grip (see Figure 20.3)
- flexion and extension of elbows
- put hands behind head.

Is there full range of movement? Is the patient in pain?

Legs

Lie the patient on a couch.
Observe for wasting, foot deformities, swellings.
Ask the patient to bend the knees up.

Hip internal rotation: with the knee bent, hold the knee and hip at 90° and gently rotate the hip internally (by pulling the foot outwards). Full range of movement? Discomfort?

Knee palpation: put the feet down on the couch. Palpate for any crepitus, warmth and swelling.

Spine

Keep the patient seated.

Lateral neck flexion: ask them to bring their ears towards their shoulders.

Stand the patient up. Inspect:

- from the sides for kyphosis
- from the back for scoliosis.

Spinal flexion and extension: ask the patient to bend forward to touch their toes and then straighten up again. Is the movement smooth and symmetrical?

Palpate for lumbar excursion. Before the patient bends down, use your fingers to mark two bony points on the lumbar spine 10 cm apart. They should separate by >5 cm as the patient bends down. Otherwise, the bending motion is happening mainly on the hip joint.

Finally

Thank the patient and allow them to get dressed in private.

Cerebellar function

Please test the patient's cerebellar function:

Cerebellar dysfunction is manifested in many ways apart from imbalance. Start with testing the head first, then gait, before proceeding to the upper and lower limbs.

1) General Observation
2) Eye movements (for nystagmus)
3) Dysarthria
4) Cerebellar Gait – unsteadiness regardless if the patient has his eyes closed or open (do not confuse this with Romberg's sign – increased unsteadiness with the eyes closed, which is indicative of sensory ataxia)
5) Hypotonia
6) Pendular reflexes
7) Incoordination
   - Finger nose test – intentional tremor
   - Dysdiadochokinesia

20 Examination of the limbs

An overview of testing the limbs

General points on technique

Be clear about the *order* of testing. Exposure and position, inspection, tone, power, reflex, co-ordination, sensation.

Test the left and right limbs separately, but to aid comparison, *test equivalent parts of each limb successively.*

Give positive commands when testing power: 'lift your leg up' instead of 'try to resist me pushing your leg down'.

Avoid repetitions. Hit the tendon *once or twice* with the tendon hammer. Likewise with moving the limbs in testing tone or touching the skin while testing sensation. Repetitions make you look unsure about your findings.

How to test tone

Before you start, get the patient to relax their weight. Saying 'Relax!' will most definitely cause the opposite effect. Instead, say 'I want you to let your arm/leg go completely floppy. Let me take your weight *(for arm)*/let it sink into the bed *(for leg)*'. Ask about pain before even touching the patient.

Describing tone

Tone can be increased (hypertonia) or decreased (hypotonia or flaccidity). Hypertonia can be further differentiated into rigidity and spasticity.

- Rigidity: increased tone throughout the range of passive movement, like a lead pipe. It is indicative of an extrapyramidal lesion and the term is used synonymously with parkinsonism.
- Spasticity: increased tone in the initial range of passive movement, leading to a sudden give, like a clasp-knife. This is indicative of and synonymous with a pyramidal/upper motor neurone lesion, typically a stroke.

Grading muscle power (MRC Scale)

Grade 0: No movement at all.
Grade 1: Flicker of movement.
Grade 2: Able to move but unable to counter gravity.
Grade 3: Able to counter gravity but not resistance.
Grade 4: Able to move against resistance.
Grade 5: Full power.

Learn this grading system as you will be expected to use it as a qualified doctor. However, in an OSCE, stick to general descriptions (see below).

Patterns of muscle weakness and common causes

Pyramidal weakness

Weakness of upper limb extensors and lower limb flexors.
Causes: upper motor neurone (UMN) lesion (e.g. stroke).

Proximal weakness

Causes: peripheral neuropathies (e.g. Guillain–Barré syndrome, diabetic neuropathy) which can be associated with sensory loss as well.

TABLE 20.1   Distinguishing an upper motor neurone (UMN) lesion from a lower motor neurone (LMN) lesion

	UMN	LMN
Tone	Increased (spastic/rigid)	Reduced
Power	Reduced	Reduced
	Pyramidal weakness	
Reflex	Increased	Absent

Generalized weakness

Causes: myasthenia gravis (muscle fatiguability, cranial nerve signs, such as facial, extraocular and bulbar weakness).

How to test reflexes

See page 152 on individual reflexes.
Only test reflexes with a tendon hammer and nothing else!
Aim for the *tendon*, not the bone or surrounding muscle. It is useful to feel the tendon before you tap it.
Learn the root value of the reflexes.

Reinforcement

If there is no response, ask the patient to do the following at the same moment you test the reflex:

● Upper limb reflex: clench their teeth.
● Lower limb reflex: lock the hands together and pull.

How to test sensation

Sensory loss is considered a 'soft' sign in neurology. In an OSCE, marks are therefore given for demonstrating good technique rather than accurate mapping of an area of sensory loss.

● Start with a clear explanation and demonstration to the patient (see below).
● Learn the dermatomes for the upper and lower limbs and test ONE spot in each dermatome. This is a good way of testing the whole limb and it also demonstrates your knowledge to the examiner. You will look far more confident than the random tester.
● Start distally then move proximally.
● Start from an area of altered sensation (if the history indicates so).
● Compare equivalent areas on the contralateral limb.
● There are five modalities of sensation: pinprick, temperature, light touch, vibration sense and proprioception. Temperature sense is rarely tested in an exam. Learn to test all four other modalities but, in an OSCE, find out what is expected by reading the instructions or asking the examiner. Do not spend all the allocated time testing just one modality.

Tools

- Light touch: cotton wool/ tissue paper.
- Pinprick: neuropins (not needles!); dispose into sharps bin after use.
- Vibration sense: tuning fork.
- Temperature: use a tuning fork and ask if the patient can feel its coolness against their skin.

Remember to *touch, not scratch* the skin with the tools, as that creates an alternative sensation of itch.

Explanation and demonstration

Before testing each sensory modality, demonstrate on a patch of skin on the chest, such as over the sternum, to ensure the patient understands what to do.

'I am going to test your sensation with this piece of cotton wool/pin/tuning fork.'

For light touch, ask 'Can you feel the cotton wool/tissue? Afterwards, I want you to *say "Yes"* every time you feel me touch you'.

For pinprick, touch the skin with the blunt end of the neuropin, explaining 'This is blunt', then with the pin 'and this is sharp. Can you feel the difference? Afterwards, I want you to tell me whether the touch is blunt or sharp'.

For vibration sense, rest an activated tuning fork on the sternum and say 'Can you feel the buzzing? Afterwards, *say "Yes"* every time you can feel the buzzing'. It is the buzzing, not the touch or even the coolness of the tuning fork, that we are interested in. Instead of testing skin, remember to rest the fork over *bone*, starting distally.

For proprioception, first explain 'I'm about to move the tip of your toe/finger either up or down'. Hold the digit just below the most distal joint (distal interphalangeal or intermetatarsal joints) and the tip of the digit with the other hand. Move the tip of the digit in one small movement and ask 'Have I moved it *up* or *down*?'. Make sure you hold the digit by its sides, not by the nail, otherwise the patient can sense the movement from the pressure on their nails.

The actual test

1. Ask the patient to *close their eyes* first, so they cannot see you touch them.
2. Test light touch in a dermatomal fashion.
3. Test pinprick in a dermatomal fashion.
4. Test proprioception, moving from small to large joints.
5. Test vibration sense, moving from small to large joints.

In an OSCE, you are likely to get two scenarios:

- glove and stocking sensory loss
- Multiple Sclerosis.

Upper limb examination

- Positioning and exposure
- General observation
- Tone
- Upper arm drift
- Power
- Reflex
- Coordination
- Sensation

Positioning and exposure

Remember to expose the whole arm, including the shoulder. If the patient is wearing a bulky jumper with long sleeves, it is reasonable to ask them to remove it.

General observation

- Wasting
- Fasciculations
- Scars
- Abnormal movements (tremors, chorea)

Be seen to inspect along the *whole length* of the limb from the shoulder and arm to hand. Do not forget wasting of small muscles of the hand.

Rest the patient's arm on their lap and watch for parkinsonian tremor (rest tremor/pill-rolling tremor), which occurs *at rest* by definition.

Tone

Inquire about pain before you start.

First get the patient to completely relax their weight. Support their elbow and say 'Let your arm go all floppy. Let me take your weight'.

Testing upper limb tone is not about shaking the patient's arm violently; you are testing tone in three purposeful movements. Hold the patient's hand, stabilize the shoulder and gently:

- bend the arm (flexion/extension)
- rotate the forearm (pronation and supination)
- rotate the wrist through 180°.

Upper arm drift

Ask the patient to put both arms out with the palms facing up. Ask them to close their eyes and keep their arms in the same position.

This test is often done but every candidate will give you a different answer as to what they are testing. This is because it is a four-in-one test.

1. Pyramidal weakness: the side with pyramidal weakness (see above for explanation of pyramidal weakness) will drift *down* with the palm faced down – so-called pronator drift.
2. Incoordination: the affected side will drift *upwards*.
3. Loss of proprioception: the fingers will be wriggling around.
4. Postural tremor: fine tremor due to a variety of causes: idiopathic, anxiety, hyperthyroidism, familial.

Power

Give simple, assertive instructions to patients and avoid double negatives.

The upper limb needs to be put into different postures and positions to test power, so demonstrate at each step: it will make life easier for both of you (Figure 20.1).

Shoulder abduction

Say 'Keep your arms up' as you demonstrate with your arms out like chicken wings, then put your hands on both of the patient's arms and say 'Keep your arms up'.

Shoulder adduction

Demonstrate with your 'chicken wings' tight against your body: 'Now keep your arms tightly against yourself' as you try to lift each arm outwards.

Extension

Show the patient how to put both arms in front of them like they are fending off a punch. Stabilize their shoulder with one hand and hold their wrist with the

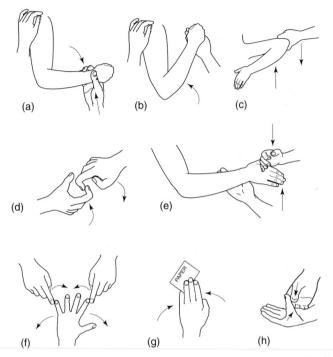

FIGURE 20.1 How to test power in the upper limbs. (a) elbow extension; (b) elbow flexion; (c) shoulder abduction; (d) finger flexion; (e) finger extension; (f) finger abduction; (g) finger adduction; (h) thumb abduction.

other hand: 'Push me away'. Make sure the forearm is at right angles to the upper arm.

Flexion

Keeping the same position, say to the patient: 'Now pull me towards you'.

Wrist flexion

Show the patient how to hold two fists out. Stabilize the forearm with one hand and rest the other hand over their wrist. Say 'Cock your wrist back'.

Finger flexion

Lock your hand into the patient's hand. Try to unravel their fist as you ask them to keep their fingers bent. Long fingernails will complicate the matter.

Finger extension

Ask the patient to slightly bend their stretched fingers at the metatarso-phalangeal joint. Hold their palm, put your hand above their outstretched fingers and ask them to push upwards.

Thumb abduction

Remember that the thumb can move in three planes: abduction/adduction, flexion/extension and opposition.

To test abduction, ask the patient to keep their palm faced up and lift the thumb up at right angles to the palm. Put your finger against the thumb and say to the patient: 'Push back against my finger'.

Reflex (Figure 20.2)

Rest the patient's arms on their lap. Ensure the cubital fossa is exposed to allow easy access to the biceps tendon.

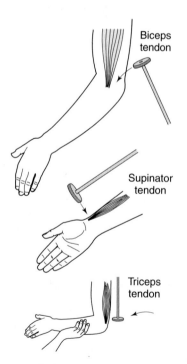

Biceps tendon

Supinator tendon

Triceps tendon

FIGURE 20.2 Reflexes in the upper limb.

Biceps jerk

Feel with two fingers for the biceps tendon and hit the tendon hammer over your fingers.

Triceps jerk

Feel for the triceps tendon and hit the hammer over your fingers.

Supinator jerk

Rotate the forearm so that the supinator tendon is facing up. Put your fingers over it and hit the tendon hammer on your fingers. Look and feel for a response.

Coordination

Do not attempt to explain the following tests to the patient in one breath. Break them down, demonstrate and encourage the patient to follow you with each step.

Hand dominance

Ask the patient whether they are right or left handed.

Finger-to-nose test

Touch the patient's index finger and say: 'I want you to use this finger to touch your nose'. Place your finger about one arm's-length away and say 'and then touch my finger here. Do it as quickly as you can'.

Get the patient used to the idea of the test and then start *moving your target*, otherwise the test is too easy and incoordination will not be elicited. Move the target when the patient is still touching their nose to give them enough time to see the target.

Be sure you comment on the *two* possible signs:

- pass-pointing (dysmetria)
- intention tremor: tremor that gets increasingly worse as it nears your target.

These are indicative of cerebellar dysfunction.

Dysdiadochokinesis

Show the patient your palm face up: say 'Put your left hand out like this, then tap your right hand on it, back and forth, as quickly as you can'. There could be a marked discrepancy between the dominant and non-dominant hand; if so, establish if the patient is right or left handed.

Sensation

See section on 'How to test sensation ' on page 139 above.

Examination of the hands

Follow the mantra of Look-Feel-Move (passive and active).

Introduction

Take a very brief history starting with name, age and occupation. Often there are specific marks for this. Enquire about pain, discomfort and take a short history regarding onset of symptoms, drug history and family history. 'Is it just your hands that are affected?'

Exposure and position

Expose the arms up to the elbows. Ask the patient to roll up their sleeves. Position the hands on the table and/or on a pillow, ensuring comfort where possible

Look at the patient. Note obvious joint deformity, tophi, rheumatoid nodule, psoriatic hairline, sticks, zimmer or wheelchair and other clues.

Look

Dorsal surface

- Scars
- Psoriatic nail changes: pitting, onycholysis
- Gout tophi: over tendons, extensor surface of forearm, also pinna of ears
- Buchard's and Heberden's nodes
- Ulnar deviation of MCPJ*
- Z-deformity of the thumb

*Abbreviations: DIPJ, distal interphalangeal joint; MCPJ, metacarpophalangeal joint; PIPJ, proximal interphalangeal joint.

Palmar surface

- Scars
- Muscle wasting: thenar eminence (median n.), hypothenar eminence (ulnar n.), anatomical snuffbox (radial n.), small muscles
- Dupuytren's contracture

Ask the patient to lift their hands. Look from the side

- Contractures
- Subluxations
- Boutonnière, swan neck deformities

Ask the patient to show you their elbows

- Rheumatoid nodules: subcutaneous, non-tender lumps. Range from 0.5 to 3 cm
- Psoriatic rash

Feel and passive movement

Undue suffering is bad and loses points, so establish with the patient what you can and cannot do and inquire about pain before you start. Look at the patient's face as you do so.

Gently squeeze each joint (wrist, MCPJ, DIPJ, PIPJ) in order; at the same time gently move it to check its range of movement.

Examine one hand at a time. Be systematic. Feel for:

- heat, dry or moist skin
- bony tenderness
- effusions
- crepitus.

Test movement for each joint.

- Wrist: flexion and extension, ulnar and radial deviation, pronation and supination
- MCP, DIP and PIP: flexion, extension

Active movement and functional grips (Figure 20.3)

Demonstrate and ask the patient to follow.
- Power grip: ask the patient to squeeze your two fingers.

(a)   (b)   (c)

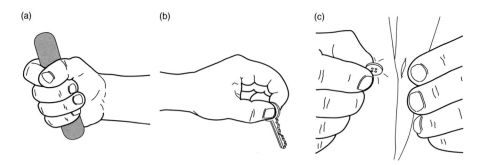

FIGURE 20.3   Function of the hand. (a) Power grip. (b) Key grip. (c) Precision grip.

- Key grip: oppose the pulps of the thumb and forefingers, like holding a key.
- Precision grip: oppose the thumb and index finger into an 'O'.

Sensation

Nerve entrapments can result from tendonitis, joint or soft tissue swelling.

Check light touch with a piece of tissue at three spots corresponding to the distribution of the median, radial, ulnar nerves (Figure 20.4), and the anatomical snuffbox.

- Tinel's test: percuss over the wrists.
- Phalen's test: ask the patient to flex their wrists for one minute.

In carpal tunnel syndrome, both tests will elicit tingling or numbness in the median nerve distribution.

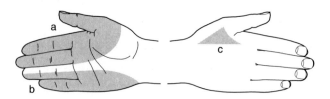

Palmar surface: a. median nerve distribution
                          b. ulnar nerve distribution
Dorsal surface: c. radial nerve distribution

FIGURE 20.4   Patterns of sensory loss in the hand.

Function

Writing with a pen
Doing up/undoing buttons

Presentation of findings

There is no need (or time) to describe each joint in turn. Learn to describe the pattern.

- Are the findings bilateral? Is it symmetrical?
- Is it a monoarthropathy or polyarthropathy?
- Comment on any diagnostic changes: swan neck, Heberden's nodes, etc.
- Comment on extra-articular signs
- Effects on function

And finally, say something intelligent! (As well as your differential!)

'I would normally perform *neurological and vascular examinations* now; would you like me to do so?'

'I would like to examine the joints in the rest of the arm/body'
and ...

'I would like to x-ray this joint/aspirate this joint/take blood for ESR, CRP, FBC, rheumatoid factor, etc ...'

When suggesting further examinations and tests, have an idea of *why* you want them, as you could be asked to explain.

What are these characteristic bony deformities?

Swan neck deformity	Hyperextension at PIPJ and fixed flexion deformity of DIPJ
Boutonnière deformity	Fixed flexion of PIPJ, extension of DIPJ
Z-deformity of thumb	Hyperextension of IPJ and fixed flexion and subluxation of MCPJ
Heberden's nodes	DIPJ swelling due to osteophytes
Bouchard's nodes	PIPJ swelling due to osteophytes

TABLE 20.2   Findings in the hands

Condition	Signs and symptoms in the hands
Rheumatoid arthritis	*Symmetrical destructive polyarthropathy* Initally: sausage-like fingers and MCPJ swelling Ulnar deviation Volar subluxation Swan neck and boutonnière deformities Z-deformity of the thumb Rheumatoid nodules Tenderness, pain on movement, stiffness
Osteoarthritis	Most commonly affects DIPJ, first MCPJ in hands Tenderness, pain at rest and on movement, stiffness Heberden's & Buchard's nodes, joint effusions Remember to think about vertebrae, hips and knees
Psoriatic arthropathy	Most commonly: monoarthropathy with sausage-like fingers Also: DIPJ arthropathy and psoriatic nail changes Similar presentation to rheumatoid Arthritis mutilans – destructive polyarthritis
Gout	Usually affects joints in the feet first; think of the big toe Unlikely to get acute gout in an OSCE. Red, hot, swollen and tender (differential is septic arthritis!) Tophi in recurrent gout ++. Look at pinnae Test: synovial fluid aspiration for microscopy, serum uric acid
Carpal tunnel syndrome	Median nerve paraesthesia Tinel's and Phalen's tests positive Wasting and weakness of small muscles along median nerve distribution
Lesions of peripheral nerves	*Median n.* 'Ape hand': LOAF – lateral two **L**umbricals, **O**PB, **A**PB, **F**PB *Radial n.* 'Drop wrist': BEST – **B**rachoradialis, **E**xtensors of wrist, **S**upinator, **T**riceps, Loss of sensation over anatomical snuffbox *Ulnar n.* 'Claw hand': MAFIA – **M**edial lumbricals ('priest's blessing' if weak), **A**dductor pollicis (pincer grip), **F**irst dorsal interossei, **I**nterossei, **A**bductor digiti minimi

Lower limb examination

- Positioning and exposure
- General observation
- Gait
- Tone
- Power
- Reflex
- Coordination
- Sensation

The biggest faux pas in lower limb testing is forgetting to test, or to mention that you will test, gait. An equally bad mistake is allowing the patient to keep their trousers and shoes on.

Position and exposure

Ask the patient to lie on a bed, with trousers, shoes and socks off. Cover the patient's waist with a towel.

General observation

- Deformities of the foot (e.g. pes cavus), abnormal posture
- Wasting
- Fasciculations
- Scars
- Abnormal movements (tremors, chorea)

Be seen to inspect along the *whole length* of the limb from the hips and thighs to lower legs and toes. Wasting is best seen in the large muscles (e.g. quadriceps) and fasciculations require a close look for several seconds for wavelike twitches. Scars of relevance are muscle or nerve biopsy, which are relatively small (<1 inch/2.5 cm).

Gait

- Observe posture
- Standing with feet together
- Standing with feet together and eyes closed (Romberg's sign)
- Short walk by the bedside
- Heel-to-toe (tightrope) walking
- Heel walking

Throughout the examination, ensure the patient does not fall: help them on and off the bed, walk *alongside* them and be heard to say 'I will catch you if you fall' to get the extra marks. See Chapter 19.

Tone

Inquire about pain before you start.

Avoid the temptation to lift the entire leg off the bed and manoeuvre it clumsily. Keep to these three simple steps instead.

1. Lift each knee off the bed gently and let go. Increased tone will cause the leg to drop heavily without much bounce.
2. Hold the knees and gently rock the legs sideways.
3. Lift the ankle off the bed and rotate it gently.

Power (Figure 20.5)

Give simple, assertive instructions to patients and avoid double negatives.

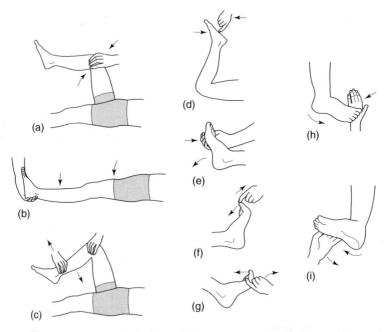

FIGURE 20.5 How to test power in the lower limb. (a) hip flexion; (b) hip extension; (c) knee flexion (reverse arrows for extension); (d) foot dorsiflexion; (e) foot plantar flexion; (f) big toe extension; (g) extension of toes; (h) foot inversion; (i) foot eversion.

To elicit full power, you need to be seen really resisting the patient, so push or pull hard against their movements (without hurting them).

Hip flexion

Say 'Lift your leg *straight* up in the air' as you push the leg down by the thigh. Make sure the knee is not bent.

Hip extension

Put your hand underneath the patient's gastrocnemius and try and lift the leg up as you say 'Push down on my hands'.

Knee extension

Ask the patient to bend both knees up. Stabilize the knee with one hand and hold the lower leg with the other. Say 'Straighten your knee and kick me away' as you push the leg in.

Knee flexion

Still stabilizing the knee, hold the ankle instead and try to pull the leg straight: '... and now pull me towards you'.

Ankle dorsiflexion

Ask the patient to straighten both legs on the bed. Hold the ankle with one hand and the entire foot with the other hand. Bend the foot down and say 'Cock your ankle back'.

Ankle plantar flexion

Still stabilizing the ankle, put one hand on the foot's plantar surface and say 'Push down on my hand' as you push their foot up.

Inversion and eversion

These two manouevres are difficult to elicit, partly because most candidates are not sure what they are.

Do the work for the patient by gently manoeuvring their foot into the everted position, if you are testing inversion, and saying 'Try and turn your foot in'. Likewise, to test eversion, put their foot in the inverted position and say 'Try and turn your foot out'.

Reflex (Figure 20.6)

Knee jerk

If the patient is lying on the bed with the legs straight, slip your hand under one knee and say 'Let me take your weight', lifting the knee off the bed slightly. Tap the patellar tendon, which is below the knee cap.

If the patient is seated, make sure their feet are off the ground and are allowed to dangle or get them to cross the leg to be tested *over* the other one.

Ankle jerk

Keep the leg straight on the bed. Place your hand on the ball of the foot and pull the foot back so that the tendon is stretched. Tap the hammer on your hand (not the patient's foot directly).

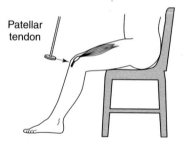

Patellar tendon

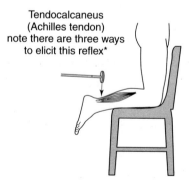

Tendocalcaneus (Achilles tendon) note there are three ways to elicit this reflex*

FIGURE 20.6   *See Fuller G., *Neurological Examination Made Easy*, 2nd Ed. p. 139, Churchill Livingstone 2000.

Babinski sign (extensor plantar reflex)

Warn the patient that you are about to scratch the sole of their foot.

Using an orange stick or the back of your thumbnail, firmly stroke the sole from the bottom, up the lateral side and across the footpad. Test both feet.

- Normal response: the foot flexes.
- Positive Babinski sign: the foot extends and the toes spread, indicative of an upper motor neurone lesion.

In many patients, even those with an UMN lesion, there may be no response or they withdraw their foot because the test is uncomfortable.

Clonus

Dorsiflex the foot sharply and maintain the position for a few seconds and the ankle will contract rhythmically. More than three beats of contractions is indicative of clonus, due to hyperreflexia.

Coordination

Explain to the patient that you are about to test his coordination. Most tests for coordination seem too bizarre otherwise.

Heel–shin test

The aim is to get the patient to run the heel down the shin of the opposite leg, then place the heel back at the top of the shin and repeat the movement. Incoordination is most obvious as the patient struggles to place the heel back on the top of the shin accurately.

This test is best explained in small steps as the patient attempts it.
'Put your right heel onto your left knee'
'... run it down your shin'
'... bring it back up to your knee'
'... then run it down the shin again. Try to do it as quickly as you can.'

Sensation

See section on 'How to test sensation' on page 139.

Examination of the knee

This is often examined as an orthopaedic station.

Inspection

Introduction

Introduce yourself and gain consent for the examination. Ask/help the patient to remove their trousers. Offer the presence of a chaperone if necessary.

Exposure and position

Always take a step back from the patient to have a good look around for clues, such as a walking stick, wheelchair or crutches.

Look

Ask the patient to stand and walk, observing:

- swelling: localized (bursa or bony overgrowth) or generalized?
- position: genu varus ('knock knees'), genu valgus ('bow legs'), fixed flexion deformity
- wasting of the quadriceps
- popliteal fossa
- gait

Feel

Ask if there is any pain/swelling. Examine the normal limb first.

Skin: warm, tender (local/general)
Effusion:

- Small
  - Patellar tap test: compress suprapatellar compartment, empty other compartments and assess for compressible patella
  - Bulge test: compress suprapatellar compartment and sweep upwards over medial compartment. Watch medial aspect for bulge as lateral compartment is compressed
- Large: loss of landmarks

Joint lines with knees flexed at 90°
Femoral condyles, patellar tendon, MCL, LCL
Popliteal fossa for swellings (Baker's cyst)
Synovial thickening
The patella itself: is it of normal shape and size? Is it tender?

Move

Active

- Flexion and extension: are these movements painful?
- Straight leg raising

Passive

- Flexion (140°): feel for crepitus and clicks
- Extension (0° to −10°)

Special tests

Collateral ligament tears (MCL and LCL)

Flex knee to 10° to relax posterior capsule (do not rotate knee).

- MCL: valgus stress in extension and flexion
- LCL: only taut in full extension and lax in flexion

Cruciate ligament tears (ACL and PCL)

Use the anterior and posterior drawer test. Place the sole of the patient's foot on the bed with knee flexed at 90° and, with permission, sit on the foot (gently). With your hands around the joint, place both thumbs over the anterior surface. Move the tibia back and forth. Does it move when you pull (ACL tear) or push (PCL tear)?

Mention the possible need to perform the following tests.

- Lachman's test (ACL tears): flex the knee to 20°. Hold the thigh with one hand, the upper calf with the other. Pull forward to test for a complete ACL tear.
- McMurray's test and Apley's grinding test (meniscal tears): these tests rely on pain to make a diagnosis, so are best left to the experts to decide when necessary. They involve holding the knee and sole of the foot and flexing whilst turning and pressing on the knee.

Extensions

Offer to perform a full distal neurovascular examination.
State that you would move on to examine both the hips and ankles of the patient. Ask for an AP and lateral x-ray of the problematic knee (MRI can be suggested).

If the knee is warm and swollen, consider the need for joint aspiration to exclude septic arthritis.

Possible OSCE stations

- Osteoarthritis: affects mainly knees and hips. Look for Heberden's (DIP) and Bouchard's (PIP) nodes on the hands. Usually bilateral. X-ray findings include: decreased joint space, osteophytes, sclerosis at joint margins and bone cysts close to joint margins.
- Baker's cyst: degenerative outpouching of the synovium in the popliteal fossa.
- Recurrent subluxation of the patella.

21 Hip

Introduction

Introduce yourself and gain consent for the examination. Ask the patient to undress down to their undergarments.

Take a step back, looking for clues (see knee examination) and ask if patient has pain in their legs? If so, which one?

Look

Standing

Inspect (from front, side and back) comparing 'normal' to affected limb for:

- wasting (quadriceps)
- scars (previous surgery)
- sinuses
- skin changes
- swelling (lipoma)
- deformity (leg length inequality, pes cavus, scoliosis)

Gait: antalgic, decreased range of movement, Trendelenburg (pelvic sway/tilt).

Trendelenburg's test

Stand the patient by a wall and ask them to stand on each leg in turn, with the other leg lifted off the ground with knee bent (Figure 21.1). Should the

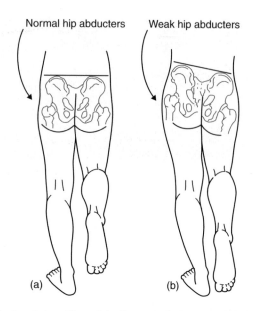

Normal hip abducters   Weak hip abducters

(a)   (b)

FIGURE 21.1   Trendelenburg's test. The pelvis tilts towards the normal hip when weight is borne.

unsupported side of the pelvis move downwards, there is an abnormal weakness of hip abductors in the stance leg (it's the sound side that sags).

Supine

Inspect again. Observe obvious limb shortening, limb rotation, abduction or adduction deformity or flexion deformity.

Measure limb length.

- True leg length: with iliac crests aligned horizontally, at 90° to trunk. Measure distance from ASIS to medial malleolus on the same side. Any shortening represents pathology of the hip joint. If there is any shortening, bend the patient's knees to 90°. Which knee is higher?
- Apparent leg length: from xiphisternum to each medial malleolus. Differences will be due to tilting of the pelvis.

Feel

Tenderness. Ask about this before touching the patient.

Skin: temperature, effusion

Anatomical landmarks: ASIS, greater trochanter, inguinal ligament

Move

Flexion

Both hips should flex to 130°.

Thomas' test

Hold one hip flexed, straighten the other leg. Keep one hand on the small of the back. Note that this abolishes the lumbar lordosis. The test is positive if the patient cannot straighten their leg – they have a fixed flexion deformity.

Abduction and adduction

With one leg over the edge of the couch and one hand on the ASIS to fix the pelvis, abduct (normal range 50°) and adduct (45°) each leg in turn.

Rotation

Flex hip and knee. Hold knee in the left hand and ankle in right hand. Bring each ankle in laterally (*internal rotation*, 45°) and medially (*external rotation*, 45°).

Prone

Look, feel, move. Extension with one hand on the sacroiliac joint and the other elevating the leg (30°).

Extensions

Offer to perform a full distal neurovascular examination of both legs.
'I would normally perform an examination of the *spine and knees*. Would you like me to do so?'
Ask for an AP and lateral x-ray of the affected hip.

Possible OSCE stations

- Osteoarthritis
- Total hip replacement (THR)
- Arthrodesis
- Slipped upper femoral epiphysis (SUFE)

Spine

Introduction

Always take a brief history. Often there are specific marks for this. Enquire about pain, neurological symptoms, such as sphincter control, and mobility.

Expose the patient adequately, with permission. As before, look for clues such as a stick or brace.

Look

- Side: lordosis and kyphosis (osteoporosis)
- Behind: scoliosis in trauma, vertebral body disease, developmental abnormalities, muscle problems

Feel

- Ask about pain/tenderness beforehand
- Spinous processes: tender in metastatic cancer, infection and collapse
- Interspinous ligaments
- Sacroiliac joints: tender in seronegative arthropathy

Move

- Gait: stand on toes and heels

- Neck: flexion, extension, lateral flexion, rotation
- Spine (hands on patient's hips): flexion, extension, lateral flexion, rotation

Perform *Schobers test*:

- Patient stands straight
- Identify PSIS and mark midline points 5 cm below and 10 cm above
- Flex spine ('Try to touch toes')
- Measure distance (start at 15 cm: should increase to >20 cm if normal, <20 cm indicates a decreased ROM, which can indicate ankylosing spondylitis)

Lie patient supine

Perform *straight leg raising test*

- Pain in thigh, buttock, back can indicate sciatica (L3, 4, 5)
- If positive, perform *Bragard's test*
- Concomitant dorsiflexion increases intensity of pain

Turn patient prone

Perform *femoral stretch test*

- Flex knee
- Extend hip
- Pain in front of thigh indicates involvement of L1 and L2

'I would normally perform *neurological and vascular examinations* now; would you like me to do so?'

Extensions

- Imaging: x-ray, MRI
- Bloods: FBC, U+Es, bone profile, ESR/CRP, electrophoresis
- Urine: Bence–Jones protein (if suspicion of myeloma)

Possible OSCE stations

Ankylosing spondylitis

- ↓ Lordosis, ↑ kyphosis
- ↓ Spinal flexion
- Apical lung fibrosis; aortic incompetence; acute iritis

Osteoarthritis

- Also examine hip and knee

Scoliosis

- Trauma
- Vertebral body disease
- Developmental disorders
- Muscle problems

Muscular back pain

- Young patient

Prolapsed intervertebral disc

- Young (if older, probably compression by osteophytes)
- Lumbago and sciatica
- Rx: mattress, analgesia, epidural corticosteroids

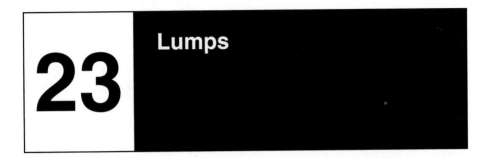

23 Lumps

These are an exam staple. Beware the person with a ping-pong ball taped to their shoulder when a real patient fails to attend. In this scenario you are expected to demonstrate what you would do without the prompt of real pathology. Treat it as real!

Always introduce yourself to the patient and obtain consent to examine. Expose the patient adequately, maintaining their dignity.

As with all examinations, it is useful to start with a few pertinent questions (if permitted):

- How long have you had this lump?
- Have you or anyone else noticed a change in the appearance of the lump?
- Is it painful?
- Have you noticed any other lumps?
- Are you otherwise well?

Examination largely involves observation and palpation. Enquire about pain/tenderness before any examination. Consider the following.

- Site/position in relation to anatomical landmarks, preferably bony structures
- Size (diameter in centimetres)
- Shape (e.g. hemispherical)
- Surface (describe the overlying skin, e.g. rough, smooth, etc.)
- Colour, e.g. is it red and inflamed?
- Consistency (e.g. hard/soft, etc.)
- Compressibility
- Temperature (compared with another part of the patient, inflammatory)
- Tenderness on palpation of the lump (inflammatory)

- Transillumination (darken the room and put a pen torch against the lump; fluid transilluminates)
- Is the lump pulsatile? (vascular)
- If so, are there any bruits in the lump on auscultation?
- Does coughing send an impulse through the lump (such as with an abdominal/scrotal hernia)?
- What is the lump's relation to deep and superficial structures? You can test this by getting the patient to tense their muscles in the relevant area and trying to pinch the skin over the lump.
- Lymph nodes are extremely important; check the regional lymph nodes (Figure 23.1) as these may indicate infection or cancer.

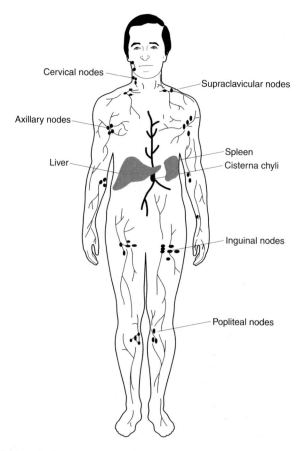

FIGURE 23.1   The lymphatic system.

Offer to help the patient re-dress and say 'Thank you', as for any examination.

Remember this system and you will not fail ... describe the lump in terms of these characteristics. The perfect description should allow someone who has never seen the patient to gain a good idea of the lump and formulate a provisional diagnosis. Suggest a diagnosis and a differential, e.g. lipoma for liposarcoma, remembering that common things are so-called because they are common. Confirmation will usually involve radiology and histology, i.e. ultrasound and biopsy. Management involves either watchful waiting, surgical removal or medication including chemotherapy (if a malignancy).

Examination of the neck/thyroid

This may well start as a neck examination but, if there is a suspicion of altered thyroid status, the onus is on you to check for peripheral thyroid signs. If you suspect a diagnosis then there may be no harm* in asking a few questions about how long a neck sign has been present, what problems it causes, and any relevant systemic features of thyroid disease, etc.

Introduction

Introduce yourself and explain the examination. Ask the patient if the lump is painful and if it has changed size.

Exposure and position

Ask the patient to unbutton his top to expose the neck down to the sternal notch. Make sure he is seated comfortably.

General inspection (from the front and the side)

- Patient: is he thyrotoxic (thin, lid retraction, proptosis, ophthalmoplegia) or hypothyroid (dry hair and skin, puffy face, pretibial myxoedema)?
- Asymmetry of neck
- Scars
- Neck lumps

*... and even some marks – check the breakdown of skills if one is available at the entrance to the station.

Midline: thyroid gland (goitre, carcinoma, adenoma) thyroglossal cyst
Anterior angle: pharyngeal pouch, carotid artery aneurysm/tumour, lymph nodes
Posterior angle: cystic hygroma, lymph nodes
Submandibular: salivary gland

- Tongue protrusion: 'Stick your tongue out please'. A thyroglossal cyst will move upwards.
- Swallow test: ask for a glass of water. 'Please sip this water, hold it in your mouth, and now swallow.' If the lump rises on swallowing, check for goitre, thyroglossal cyst, lymph nodes.

Palpation

From in front
'I am now going to gently feel your neck. Is that all right?'

- Feel the lump(s) for size, shape, constituency and mobility
- Check for transillumination: cystic hygroma, thyroglossal cyst
- Feel for tracheal deviation

Stand behind the patient

- Palpate the lump from behind
- Repeat swallow test: 'Can I get you to drink a sip of water again while I examine the lump?' Palpate the lump as the patient swallows
- Lymph nodes: supraclavicular fossae, cervical chain, submandibular and submental
- Proptosis: while standing behind, look from the top for proptosis.

Percussion

- Retrosternal extension: percuss over the manubrium from right to left. Dullness could indicate a retrosternal extension of a goitre.

Auscultation of lump

- Bruit: thyrotoxicosis.

Extensions

If thyrotoxic

- Heat intolerance

- Anxiety
- Hands: warm, tremor, onycholysis, thyroid acropachy, palmar erythema
- Eyes: lid retraction, lid lag, proptosis, ophthalmoplegia
- CVS: AF, tachycardia
- CNS: proximal myopathy
- Dermatology: pretibial myxoedema
- Treatment: propanolol, carbimazole, radioactive iodine, thyroidectomy

If hypothyroid

- History of weight gain, cold intolerance and/or constipation
- Speech: croaking, cognitive slowness
- CVS: bradycardia
- CNS: delayed relaxation of ankle jerks
- Dermatology: cool, dry skin; alopecia and thinning of scalp hair
- Treatment: thyroxine

Investigations

- TFTs
- Thyroid autoantibodies
- Ultrasound scan of neck/thyroid
- Iodine thyroid scan
- FNAC

Part 5

Special situations

Basic information

Age, occupation.

Presenting complaint

Menorrhagia

- Duration of problem?
- Assess blood loss: frequency of changing tampons, soiled underwear, flooding, passage of clots.
- Prolonged periods? (fibroids)
- Dysmenorrhoea? (endometriosis, fibroids)
- Dyspareunia? (endometriosis)
- Intermenstrual bleed? (endometrial carcinoma)
- Regularity of cycles?
- Use of intrauterine coil?
- Anaemia: fatigue, breathlessness?
- Blood dyscrasia: 'Do you bruise easily?' 'If you cut yourself, do you stop bleeding quickly?'
- History and symptoms of hypo/hyperthyroidism?
- Effects on daily life?
- Previous investigations/treatments?

TABLE 25.1   Causes of menorrhagia and their associated features

Cause	Features
Fibroids	Regular, painful, heavy periods
Endometrial Polyps	Prolonged periods
Endometriosis	Regular, painful, heavy periods
	Pelvic pain (dysmenorrhoea or dyspareunia) is the main complaint
Dysfunctional uterine bleeding (*a term used when no pathological cause is found*)	Heavy periods with no other symptoms
Intrauterine coil	Dysmenorrhoea
Endometrial carcinoma	Intermenstrual bleed
Thyroid disorders	Irregular cycles

Postmenopausal bleeding

- Duration of symptoms
- Last menstrual period
- Pattern of blood loss: how many days each time? Frequency?
- On HRT: what type?
- Assess blood loss: spotting or similar amount to a period?
- Any blood-stained, watery vaginal discharge?
- Previous smear test and results
- Superficial dyspareunia, vulval soreness

TABLE 25.2   Causes of postmenopausal bleeding and associated features

Cause	Features
Atrophic vaginitis	Superficial dyspareunia, vulval soreness
HRT-related withdrawal bleed	
Endometrial carcinoma	Watery, blood-stained discharge
Cervical carcinoma	Watery, blood-stained discharge
	History of sexually transmitted diseases
	History of abnormal smear test

Acute pelvic pain

- Site of pain: lower abdominal/iliac fossa/referred to shoulder tip? Unilateral or bilateral?
- Pyrexia
- Last menstrual period
- Irregular periods

- Vaginal discharge: thick, yellow, offensive smelling
- History of STDs

TABLE 25.3   Causes of acute pelvic pain

Cause	Features
Acute salpingitis	Throbbing lower abdominal pain, bilateral fever, abnormal vaginal discharge
Ectopic pregnancy	Acute, severe pain, referred to shoulder Vaginal bleeding History of irregular periods increases risk
Ruptured ovarian cyst	Acute abdominal pain, more on one side
Mid-cycle pain/ovulation	Aching pain in iliac fossa
Ovarian torsion	Sudden acute lower abdominal pain, localized to unilateral iliac fossa
Non-gynaecological causes	

Chronic pelvic pain

- Cyclical or constant?
- Deep dyspareunia
- Backache in the sacral region
- Thick, yellowy, offensive-smelling vaginal discharge?
- Dysmenorrhoea
- Menorrhagia
- Previous sexually transmitted diseases?
- Previous pelvic surgery
- Use of analgesia
- Bowel symptoms (irritable bowel)

TABLE 25.4   Causes of chronic pelvic pain

Cause	Features
Endometriosis	Cyclical pain Dyspareunia Regular, heavy, painful periods
Pelvic inflammatory disease	Constant pain Dyspareunia Backache referred to the sacral region Heavy, painful periods Malodorous, thick vaginal discharge History of STDs
Adhesions	Previous pelvic surgery

Dyspareunia (pain during intercourse)

- Deep (endometriosis, fibroids, ovarian cyst, PID, adhesions, vaginal stenosis, psychogenic vaginismus) or superficial (atrophic vaginitis, vulval dystrophy, vaginal scarring)?
- Chronic pelvic pain?
- Menorrhagia (fibroids, PID)
- Effects on patient's relationship with partner, emotional effects

Past obstetric and gynaecological history

Including investigations, medical and surgical treatment.

Menstrual history

- Regularity of periods
- Duration of each cycle, number of days of bleeding
- Dysmenorrhoea: painful periods?
- Menorrhagia
- Intermenstrual bleed

If the patient is in the menopausal age range (40+), elicit this tactfully: 'When was your last period?'.

For postmenopausal women, ask about postmenopausal bleeding.

Cervical smears

- Time lapse from last smear test and results
- Previous abnormal tests
- Treatment

Sexual function and contraception

- Are you currently sexually active?
- Are you using any contraception? What are you using?
- Have you tried other forms of contraception before?
- Dyspareunia: deep/superficial

Past medical history

- Include bowel and bladder function
- Thrombosis

Drug and allergy history

For example, any medicine that could prolong bleeding.

Family history

- Cancers of the breast, colon or ovary
- Thrombosis, strokes

Social history

This may reveal risk factors for genitourinary disease.

Sexually transmitted diseases and HIV

Scenario 1

George, a 35-year-old man, has presented to the genitourinary walk-in clinic. He is worried because he is experiencing some urethral discharge and burning.

Introduction

Hello George, I'm Dr Jane Smith. What prompted you to come here today? What do you think might be causing these problems? Why do you think you have a sexually transmitted disease?

Presenting complaint

Onset and duration of symptoms
Discharge: amount, smell, colour
Dysuria, urinary urgency
Painful genital rash (?herpes)
Fever
Joint pain

Sexual history

'I need to ask you some personal questions about your sexual health. Are you sexually active currently? (If not, have you been sexually active in the past?) Does your partner experience the same symptoms?'

Number of current partners
Male or female?
Sex abroad?
Last sexual intercourse
'Do you practise vaginal sex, oral sex, anal sex?'
Method of contraception
Use of condoms
Previous sexually transmitted disease and treatment

Medical and drug history

Social history

Occupation
Smoking, alcohol and recreational drugs

Explanation and education

Need for a urethral swab
Tests for chlamydia, gonorrhoea, syphilis
Results in one hour
Encourage discussion with partners and get them tested – women risk
    infertility
Contact slip for partners
Confidentiality
Educate about safe sex

Scenario 2

David is currently an inpatient with a severe chest infection. The pathogen has
been confirmed as *Pneumocystis carinii*. You are here to discuss the findings
and request an HIV test.

Introduction

Hello David, I'm Dr Jane Smith. I've come to discuss with you a few issues
about your chest infection.

Broaching the subject

'The test from the laboratory grew a bug called PCP.'
'This type of infection usually happens in people whose immune system is weak.'
'One of these reasons could be HIV infection.'
'Do you think you could be HIV positive?'
'As you might know, HIV is transmitted usually by sexual intercourse. Do you
   mind if I ask you a few personal questions about your sexual health?'

Sexual history (see above)

Have you *ever* had unprotected sexual intercourse... etc.

Other risk factors

Previous blood transfusions?
'Have you ever used any illicit drugs?'
'What do you use?'
'Do you inject?'
'Do you share needles?'

Explain HIV test

HIV is the virus that causes AIDS.
Strongly advise the patient to undergo the test as it is indicated in this case.
A simple blood test.
Results take several days.
Confidential, will not be divulged to your GP if you specify.
Requires written consent.

What if it is positive?

'There is no cure as yet for HIV but there is treatment to control the disease
   and slow its progression'.
Antiretroviral treatment
Refer to specialist team for your care
Improved treatment means longer life expectancy

Summarize

'I can understand you are nervous and worried. Would you like to talk to a
   counsellor?'

Offer information leaflet

Give patient time to think and make a decision. Offer to come back later

Reassure about confidentiality

Communication

- Broach the subjects of STD/HIV carefully.
- Be non-judgmental, supportive and sympathetic.
- Be honest. Do not give patient false reassurance (e.g. I'm sure your test will be fine.').
- Be informative and helpful.
- Confidentiality (see Chapter 3 on ethics).

---

27 Oral contraceptive pill and emergency contraception

ORAL CONTRACEPTION

> **Scenario 1**
>
> You are a GP and a young lady in her 20s attends your practice as she would like to start the oral contraceptive pill.

Introduction

'Good afternoon. I'm Dr Jane Smith. I understand you want to talk about contraception. How can I help?'

Explore ideas and understanding

Why does she want to start the oral contraceptive?
Is she having problems with her current method?

Brief sexual history

'Are you currently sexually active?'
'Are you using any contraception?'
'What type?'
'Do you use it every time (for barrier methods)?'
Problems with current method?

Brief O&G history

Menstrual history
Previous sexually transmitted diseases
Obstetrics history

Brief medical history

Relative contraindications to the pill: thromboses, clotting tendency, smoker, over 35 years of age, migraine, strong family history of thromboses. Pregnancy is an absolute contraindication.

Drug history

Medication that reduces efficacy of pill: anticonvulsants, rifampicin

Oral contraceptive pill

Mechanism

Two types (combined and progesterone only) with different hormones
Downregulates hormones so ovaries do not release an egg or prevents sperm entering the womb
Does not prevent sexually transmitted diseases

Method

Once daily for 21 days then one-week break
Withdrawal bleed
Vomiting or antibiotic use reduces efficacy – use condoms for seven days

Efficacy

99% *if taken correctly.* Need to remember daily to take it! There is a twelve hour window for a 'missed pill'.
Stress her responsibilities

Disadvantages

Increases the risk of arterial and venous thromboses (DVT, strokes, MI)
Increases risk of death if age >40 or smoker
Breast tenderness

Advantages

Lighter, regular, less painful periods
Reduces risk of endometriosis, endometrial carcinoma, ovarian tumours

Suggest alternative forms of contraception

If the pill is contraindicated or the patient does not seem to be responsible/ sensible enough to handle it, suggest other types of contraception.
Explain why the oral contraceptive pill is unsuitable and suggest other methods.
Come to an agreed plan.

Summary

Check patient's understanding
Encourage questions
Give the patient an information leaflet

Communication hints

- Sensitive handling of issues
- Be personable
- Deal with patient's embarrassment sensitively
- Explore patient's ideas and concerns
- Be informative
- Be objective – allow patient to make her own decision

Other possible OSCE stations

- Depot hormonal implant
- Intrauterine device
- Explain/demonstrate how to use the condom

Emergency contraception

Scenario 2

Emma, who is 15 years old, has come to A&E in a panic. She says her contraception has failed and is seeking emergency contraception.

Introduction

'Hello, Emma, I'm Dr Jane Smith. I understand you are very upset and worried but let's sit down and go through the details and see what we can do. Tell me what's been happening.'

Presenting complaint

Time of last sexual intercourse (days/hours ago)?
Ensure it was penetrative intercourse
Any contraception used?
How did it fail: missed pill/split condom?
Has this happened before?
Is there a chance you could be pregnant?
Last menstrual period?
Regularity of cycles?

Brief O&G and medical, drug and allergy history

Cautions: previous ectopic pregnancy, liver disease
Contraindication: porphyria

Oral emergency contraception

Works by making it difficult for an embryo to implant into the womb
Should be taken within 72 hours of intercourse
'Take the two tablets as soon as possible' (previously the advice was to take them 12 hours apart)
The earlier it is taken, the more effective it is, but efficacy is not guaranteed
Side-effects usually mild, e.g. vomiting
If vomiting occurs within three hours, a replacement dose is needed
It is not acceptable as the usual form of contraception
Recommend a pregnancy test before prescribing this.

Warning

The next period could be delayed or early
You should see a doctor for a pregnancy test if the next period is late
A condom is needed till the next period
See a doctor urgently if you develop lower abdominal pain (ectopic pregnancy)

Alternative option – intrauterine device

Can be used up to 120 hours after intercourse
More effective than oral emergency contraception
More invasive

Prevention of future failures

Educate about the need for contraception and safe sex
Demonstrate how to use a condom
Tips to help patient remember to take the pill
Discuss alternative forms of contraception if necessary
Stress her responsibility

Check understanding and competence

For under 16-year-olds, the emergency pill cannot be given without parental consent unless you think the child is competent. 'Do you understand what we've discussed? Are you sure? Would you like to speak to your parents first?'

Summary

Summarize
Encourage questions
Give the patient information leaflets

Communication

- Be non-judgmental and sympathetic
- Be calming and supportive
- Listen to the patient's concerns and fears
- Take the opportunity to educate

28

Vaginal examination and cervical smear and swab

In real life, these would be performed in the following order: 1. Abdominal Exam, 2. Speculum, 3. Vaginal examination.

Vaginal examination

If you are male, make sure you are accompanied by a female chaperone, usually another healthcare professional.

If a smear test or endocervical swab is needed, it should be done before a vaginal examination.

Ask the patient to empty her bladder first, as a full bladder can conceal the vagina.

Explanation and consent

'Hello, I'm Jane Smith, one of the doctors here. Is it all right if I perform an internal vaginal examination? It should not be painful but will mainly be uncomfortable. Sister Smith will be present as well. Have you emptied your bladder yet?'

Position and exposure

Ensure privacy. Lie the patient flat. Ask her to remove her underwear. Expose below the costal margins downwards but cover her pelvic region with a towel.

Abdominal examination

Always remember to perform an abdominal examination first.

Reposition patient for vaginal exam

Ask the patient to draw her knees up and let them flop out. Keep the towel over her pelvis.

General inspection

Put a glove on your right hand. Then check for vulval swelling, inflammation, ulceration, discharge, prolapse.

Bimanual vaginal examination

Lubricate your right-hand fingers with some KY jelly. Warn the patient: 'I'm going to start the internal examination now. Let me know if I'm causing you any pain'. Observe the patient's face for pain at all times.

Part the labia with the fingers of your left hand. Insert your right index finger gently into the vagina, aiming upwards at 45°.

1. Assess with your internal finger:
   - vaginal wall: masses, foreign body
   - cervix: consistency (any tears, ulcerations), tenderness (cervical excitation), os (should be closed).
2. Place your left hand just below the patient's umbilicus for bimanual examination. Catch the uterus between your left hand and internal finger and assess for:
   - size
   - consistency (firm/hard)
   - direction (anteverted: can be palpated between the two hands; retroverted in 20% of women: can only be palpated from the pouch of Douglas)
   - mobility
   - masses
   - tenderness.
3. Shift the internal finger into the right lateral fornix and the left hand follows it to the right iliac fossa.
   - fallopian tube: it cannot be felt normally unless it's thickened
   - ovary (small mobile structure): tenderness, masses (rarely felt).

Repeat for the left fornix.

4. Now pass the finger into the posterior fornix to detect any swelling, tenderness or tethering in the pouch of Douglas.
5. Withdraw the right index finger and check it for bleeding and discharge.

Finally

Let the patient get dressed in private. Wash your hands and present your findings.

Cervical smear and endocervical swab (done prior to vaginal examination)

Equipment needed

- Cusco (bivalve) speculum (Figure 28.1a)
- Ayres spatula (Figure 28.1b)
- KY jelly
- Fixative spray
- Microscope slides
- Bright lamp

(a)

(b)

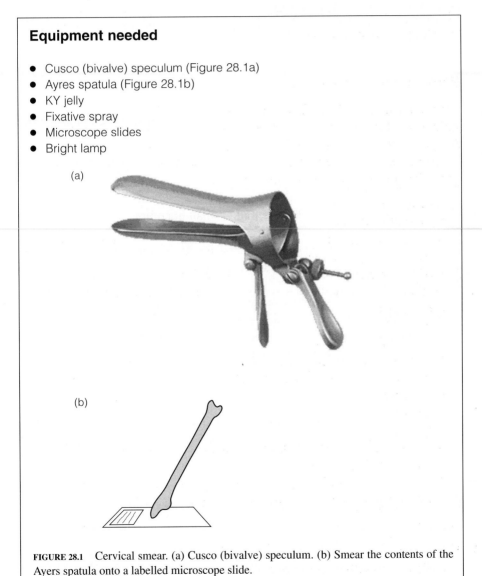

FIGURE 28.1   Cervical smear. (a) Cusco (bivalve) speculum. (b) Smear the contents of the Ayers spatula onto a labelled microscope slide.

Introduction and explanation

'Good afternoon. I'm Jane Smith and I'm one of the doctors here. I'm going to perform a cervical smear test and also take a swab. Have you had one done before?

The reason for doing the smear test is to check for any abnormal cells on the neck of the womb, which might need treating.

I will insert a speculum into the vagina and gently sweep the surface of the neck of the womb with a wooden spatula.

This should not be painful but it might be a little uncomfortable. Are you ready? Do you have any questions?'

Position and exposure

Lie the patient flat on the couch. Ask her to remove her underwear. 'Draw your knees up. Keep your feet together and just let your knees flop outwards.' Position a bright lamp to aid the visualization of the cervix later.

Prepare the speculum

Choose an appropriately sized speculum – small, medium, or large; medium is usually suitable. Remove its wrapper.

Warm the speculum in warm water – this is a kind option but you will not be expected to do so in an exam due to time constraints. Assemble the speculum by flipping the clasp.

Squirt some KY jelly onto a piece of paper towel and smear some on the speculum. Also get ready a wooden smear stick (Ayre's spatula).

When both a cervical smear and endocervical swab are needed, the swab is done last to reduce disruption to the cervical cells.

Label the slides

Using a pencil, write on the frosted end of a microscope slide: patient's name, date of birth, hospital number, date of examination, and specimen: Cervical smear.

Do not forget handwashing and gloves

Insert the speculum

'I'm about to insert the speculum now. Are you OK?'

Use your left hand to part the labia, your right hand to hold the speculum.

Ensure the speculum is closed before insertion to prevent catching on the vaginal wall. Insert it sideways, slowly. Rotate it so that the clasp is at 12 o'clock.

Gently open the speculum and lock it by turning the screw on the clasp.

Taking the smear

Look and identify the cervical os. Insert the Ayres spatula into the cervical os and twirl it around 360°.

Smear the contents onto the prepared slide (see Figure 28.1b). Spray some fixative on the slide.

Taking the endocervical swab

Insert the swab and take a sample from the *cervical os,* not the vaginal wall.

Remove the speculum

Remove the speculum under direct vision or you risk trapping the cervix.

Finally

Place the slide onto a slide holder. Fill in a histopathology request form (Figure 28.2). Label the swab sample and fill in a microbiology request form.

Allow the patient to get dressed in private. Explain that the results will be ready in a few weeks. Encourage questions.

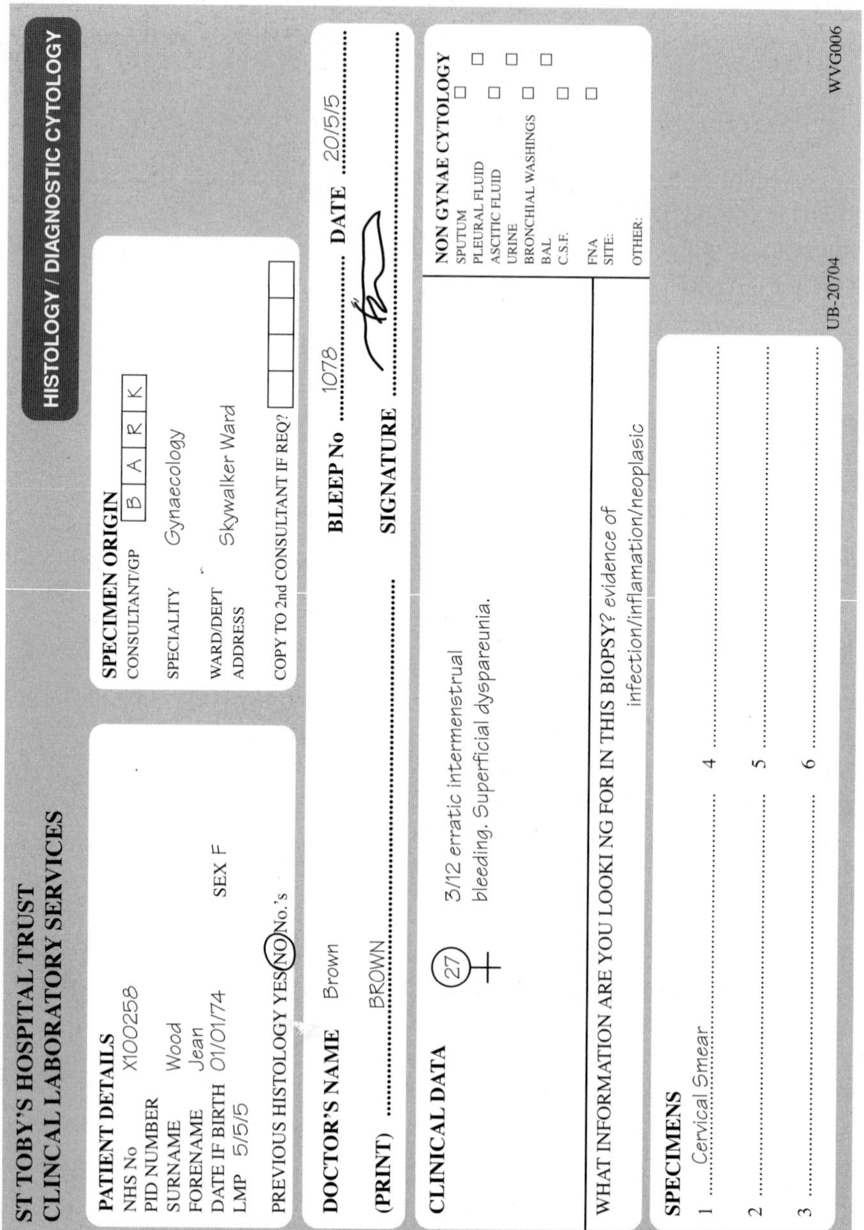

FIGURE 28.2 Example of a histopathology request form.

29

Obstetrics

Obstetrics history

Booking visit (8–12 weeks)

General information

Age? Is this your first pregnancy?

Current pregnancy

When and how was pregnancy confirmed?
First day of last menstrual period (LMP)?
Regularity of cycles. Was she taking any oral contraception?
Symptoms of pregnancy: morning sickness, urinary symptoms
Any bleeding?

Calculate expected delivery date (EDD)

- Add 9 months and 7 days to the first day of LMP, or,
- Add one year, subtract 3 months, and add 7 days.

Past obstetrics history – in chronological order

'How many times have you been pregnant before?' (miscarriages, terminations, stillbirths)
When: year?

Paternity: 'Were these pregnancies with the same partner?'
Complications: gestational diabetes, hypertension, anaemia, vaginal bleeding, abnormal scans
Outcome of pregnancies: 'Did they result in normal births?'
Deliveries:

- gestation (weeks) at birth
- sex of baby, singleton/twins
- method of delivery: spontaneous or induced? Caesarean section (why?)/ ventouse/forceps
- complications during birth
- fetal complications: 'Was the baby healthy at birth?' Birth weight?
- does he/she have any health problems now?

Gynaecological history

Last cervical smear. Results and any previous abnormal smears?

Past medical history

Diabetes, anaemia, sickle cell anaemia, hypertension, thyroid disease, epilepsy, DVT.

Drug and allergy history

Note all drugs taken in the pregnancy so far. Include analgesics, herbal and vitamin supplements.

Family history

In particular, hereditary diseases.

Social history

Marital status
Occupation
Financial support: does the partner have an income? Benefits?
Living conditions and support: 'Who do you live with?' (partner/husband/ children) 'Is there anybody to help you with the baby after you deliver?'
Alcohol intake and smoking

Summary

Encourage questions, elicit anxieties and expectations. You might be expected to discuss briefly some related topics.

- Investigations and examinations done in the booking visit:
  - general physical and breast exam (vaginal exam not usually needed)
  - urine test for glucose and protein
  - blood pressure
  - blood tests: haemoglobin, rhesus blood group, sickle screen, rubella antibodies, HIV, hepatitis test if necessary, triple test for Down's syndrome
  - need for dating (transvaginal) ultrasound if LMP is unreliable
  - CXR (history or risks of TB)
- Plans for future tests and visits
- Need for hospital booking in special circumstances
- Dietary, smoking and alcohol advice
- Social and welfare benefits

Later visits

Check for any recent events
Complications: vaginal bleeding, abdominal pain?
Common complaints: oedema, pruritus, heartburn, backache, urinary incontinence, cramps, carpal tunnel syndrome
Investigations and results so far: BP, urine dipstick for proteinuria, ultrasound scans, Down's syndrome screening
Fetal growth: movements and frequency. Ask to see the antenatal record book for: maternal weight, symphysofundal heights
Social situation: How is the mother coping? Is she still at work? Is the family supportive?
Be prepared to discuss:

- Down's syndrome screening
- amniocentesis
- chorionic villus sampling
- ultrasound scans:
  - 12 weeks: dating scan
  - nuchal scan 13–15 weeks
  - 20 weeks: anomaly scan
  - third trimester scans if complicated pregnancy
- pain relief in labour
- breast feeding

Antenatal visits

- Booking visit – weeks 8–12
- Special visits:
  13–15 weeks, nuchal scan
  16 weeks – blood test for αFP for neural tube defects
  20 weeks – anomaly scan
- 16–32 weeks – every 4 weeks
- 32–36 weeks – every 2 weeks
- 36 weeks onwards – weekly

Obstetric complications

In an OSCE station of an obstetric complication, you are most likely to be asked to take a history and suggest any suitable investigation. Physical examination is unlikely, though you might be asked about the findings for each condition. Your communication skills are particularly important in these situations.

Brief background obstetric history

Maternal age
Gestation in weeks
Number of previous pregnancies
Progress so far

Abdominal pain

Site, duration, onset
Nature of pain: comes in waves (contractions)?
Vaginal bleeding?
Systemic symptoms: vomiting, fever, symptoms of a surgical cause (e.g. appendicitis, cholecystitis)

Is this ectopic pregnancy?

Sudden-onset sharp pain or dull ache for several days are both possible
Is the pain more marked unilaterally?
Has she had an ultrasound scan to confirm intrauterine pregnancy?
Erratic menstrual cycle

Previous pelvic inflammatory disease
Previous tubal surgery
Previous ectopic pregnancy
Has intrauterine coil

Examination and investigations
Tenderness in the adnexa
βHCG raised
Transvaginal ultrasound: empty uterus

Is this a miscarriage?

Is this happening at <24 weeks?
Vaginal bleeding and passage of clots
Evidence of septic miscarriage: fever, systemically unwell, offensive vaginal
   discharge
Associated contractions: suggests inevitable miscarriage

Examination and investigations
Is the cervical os open or closed?
βHCG
Ultraound: is the fetus still present? Fetal movement? Retained products of
   conception?

Vaginal bleeding

When did this begin?
How many times has this happened? Recurrent? Stopped now?
How much bleeding: spotting? Did it soak your clothes?

TABLE 29.1   Causes of abdominal pain in pregnancy

Trimester	Cause of pain
First trimester	Ectopic pregnancy
	Miscarriage
Second trimester	Miscarriage
	Impacted retroverted uterus
Third trimester	Labour (or premature labour)
	Placental abruption
All trimesters	Surgical or medical causes, e.g. appendicitis, cholecystitis, gastroenteritis, UTI

TABLE 29.2   Signs and symptoms of miscarriage

Type	Bleeding	Abdominal pain	Os	Other findings
Threatened	Minor	Minor	Closed	Normal uterus
Inevitable	Passage of products of conception	Significant (contractions)	Open	Vasovagal attack (low pulse and BP) Large uterus
Missed	None	None	Closed	Small-for-dates uterus No fetal movement
Septic	Brown colour Offensive smell	Significant	Open	Tender, bulky uterus
Incomplete	Moderate to heavy	Significant	Open	Small-for-dates uterus
Complete	Previously	Previously	Closed	Small-for-dates uterus or cessation of all signs of pregnancy

Any clots?

Abdominal pain? How do you feel right now? (faint, breathless, chest pain – signs of shock?)

Fetal well-being: When was the last time the baby moved?

Placenta praevia

Placenta is implanted in the lower segment of the uterus:

Recurrent *painless* bright red bleeding. Only occurs after 24 weeks

Soft abdomen

Avoid digital vaginal examination

Ultrasound diagnosis: to assess position of placenta

Check haemoglobin, cross-match blood

Placental abruption

Placenta prematurely separates from the uterus before delivery:

Amount of visible blood is out of step with the degree of shock due to concealed haemorrhage

Woody hard uterus (due to tonic contraction), inability to feel fetal parts

Fetal monitoring may show signs of compromise

Check haemoglobin, clotting (risk of DIC), cross-match blood (Rhesus status)

Abdominal ultrasound may show clot behind placenta

TABLE 29.3   Causes of vaginal bleeding in pregnancy

Timing	Causes
Early	Miscarriage
	Ectopic pregnancy (main complaint is pain)
	Hydatidiform mole (bleeding without pain)
	Local causes in the vagina and cervix
Late	Placental abruption
(>24 weeks is termed	Placenta praevia (painless)
antepartum haemorrhage)	Local causes in the vagina and cervix

Examination of the pregnant abdomen

Many medical schools use a dummy gravid abdomen for this exam, which you need to treat with as much care as you would a real pregnant woman.

Introduction and explanation

'Good morning, I'm Jane Smith and I'm one of the doctors here. Is it all right for me to examine your abdomen to assess the size of the womb and also feel the position of the baby? Thank you.'

Position and exposure

Lie the mother flat on the couch with a pillow or inclined at 45°.
With permission, expose from the costal margins to the symphysis pubis.
Ensure the mother is comfortable.

Inspection

Distended abdomen
Scars (Pfannestiel scar from previous caesarean section)
Linea nigra, striae gravidarum
Fetal movements (>24 weeks)

Symphysofundal height (SFH)

Inquire about pain before you start. Palpate the abdomen from the symphysis pubis upwards until you identify the fundus. *The uterus is palpable from week 12, reaches the umbilicus by weeks 20–2 and lies under the ribs by week 36.*

Run a tape measure from the fundus down to the symphysis pubis. Measure the SFH in centimetres. Repeat once and take the average measurement.

From week 20, SFH in cm approximates to the number of gestational weeks and increases by 1 cm/week.

Palpation

Watch the patient's face for pain during the examination.
In the third trimester, assess for:

- number of fetuses
- lie: oblique, longitudinal, transverse.

From 32 weeks onwards, assess:

- presentation: cephalic/breech
- engagement: in fifths palpable.

To assess presentation and engagement, turn to face the mother's feet and palpate close to the pelvis.

Auscultation

The fetal heartbeat can be heard with Doppler ultrasound (>12 weeks) or, rarely, a Pinard stethoscope (>24 weeks). It is best heard over the fetus's anterior shoulder.

Blood pressure and urine dipsticks

To conclude, state you would like to check the mother's blood pressure and test her urine for proteinuria (pre-eclampsia) and glucose (gestational diabetes).

How to describe the fetus

Lie

Relation of the longitudinal axis of the fetus to the uterus
Described as longitudinal, transverse or oblique

Presentation

The part of the fetus in relation to the pelvic inlet

Engagement

The amount of fetal head that has entered the pelvis
Measured as fifths of fetal head palpable in the abdomen

---

30 Paediatrics

Examination of the newborn

You are unlikely to get a real baby in your OSCE so practise with a baby doll and get your monologue well rehearsed. For those who get examined by the cotside, the best time to examine a real baby is after a feed when they are content and quiet.

The general scheme is to start from the head and face and work down the body and limbs. Be opportunistic. If eyes are open check the red reflex. If baby is quiet then auscultate the chest.

Hand washing, parental permission

'Hello, my name is Jane Smith and I'm a doctor here.' First congratulate the new mother. 'Would you mind if I examine your baby? This is a routine examination we do on all newborn babies.'

Position and exposure

Start with the baby wrapped up warm in the cot or in the mother's arms. Keep him clothed initially. You will need to expose baby fully in the course of the examination.

Observe

General colour (jaundice is common in new babies), colour of lips (for cyanosis), state of alertness. Note any obvious dysmorphisms.

Fontanelles

Warm your hands before feeling the fontanelles.

● Bulging: during crying (normal), raised intracranial pressure
● Sunken: dehydration

Mouth and palate

Introduce a clean little finger into the mouth to feel for a cleft palate. You can also assess suckling at this point. If baby is crying look into the mouth for a cleft palate.

Eyes

While the baby is still warm and calm, use the ophthalmoscope to check for red reflexes.

Look for discharge from the eyes, which may indicate an infection.

Clavicles

Feel the clavicles to exclude any fractures sustained at birth, especially if you elicit an assymetrical moro reflex.

Chest

Remove the baby's clothing to expose the chest and abdomen. Observe for symmetrical chest movements and ease of respiratory effort and make sure there is no intercostal recession.

Count respiratory rate (30–50/min at rest). Listen with a stethoscope for breath sounds and for heart sounds. Check the brachial pulse (100–160/min), and listen for murmurs (innocent murmurs are Soft, Short, Sternal (L) edge, Systolic and Symptomless).

Abdomen

Observe – it is normal for the abdomen to be distended. Check the umbilicus (or cord in a newborn) for blood or discharge.

Gently palpate the four quadrants. You may feel:

● tip of the spleen
● liver edge

- both kidneys: are they enlarged?
- bladder: might cause the baby to urinate on palpation – beware. An enlarged bladder suggests urinary obstruction
- femoral pulses (radiofemoral delay suggests aortic coarctation)

Genitals

Remove the nappy and check its contents. Ask has baby passed urine and opened bowels. Examine the genitals:

- boys: exclude hernias, hydrocoeles and hypospadias. Check for symmetry of scrota, feel for both testes
- girls: exclude labial fusion.

Hips

Make sure the baby is placed on a flat surface. Be very gentle with this test. Check for hip dislocation (Ostolani and Barlow method). Babies find this test unpleasant – you may wish to leave it till last.

For Otolani's test* the baby should be placed supine on a firm surface and the hips and knees flexed to 90°. Each leg is examined in turn and is grasped with the examiner's middle finger over the greater trochanter. The thigh is lifted and gently abducted to allow a dislocated femoral head to return to the acetabulum with a notable 'clunk'. It will be noted that the femoral head moves forward if this occurs.

For Barlow's test the pelvis is fixed with one hand, placing the fingers at the back and the thumb over the symphysis pubis. The other hand is used to grip the opposite thigh and this is adducted with gentle downward pressure encouraging the femoral head to slip backwards over the lip of the acetabulum. Many paediatric departments have a 'doll' with specially made hips which can simulate the feeling of abnormal hip examinations.

Spine and anus

Pick the baby up, turn him prone and support him with your left hand. Feel the spine for scoliosis.

Check the sacral region for signs of neural tube defects such as tufts of hair, sinuses and dimples. Gently part the buttocks to check for presence of the anus. Ask if baby has had a bowel motion.

*Bellman, M. & Kennedy, N. Paediatrics and Child Health, 2000; Elsevier, Ch. 3.

Hands and feet

Count the number of digits on each hand and foot. Look out for single palmar crease, rocker-bottom feet, talipes and pedal oedema.

Neurological exam

Posture and tone are assessed thoroughout the examination. Is baby stiff or floppy? Look for abnormal repetitive movements, asymmetry of the face when crying (VIIth nerve palsy).

Tone

- Lift the baby up by the arms.
- Hold the baby prone (ventral suspension): Baby should be lifting head above midline by 4 weeks.

Moro reflex

Explain to the parents what you are about to do. Cradle the baby in your left arm and support his head in your right hand. Let the head drop. Watch the upper limbs abduct, extend and flex in a flowing movement that is symmetrical. An asymmetrical movement would make you suspicious of a clavicle fracture, Erb's palsy or other birth injury.

Grasp reflex

Place a finger across his palm and he should grasp it.

Measurements (offer to do these even if no equipment is visible)

Head circumference: measure the maximum occipitofrontal circumference.
Crown–heel length: lie the baby down for this.
Body weight: all clothing should be removed.
Plot the measurements on a centile chart.

General approach to paediatrics

Children are not little adults

- You need to adapt the physical examination routine of adults for children.

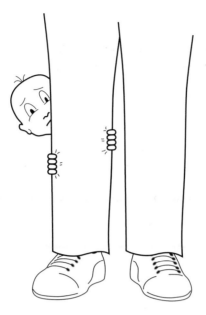

FIGURE 30.1   Children are not little adults.

- The signs and differential diagnoses are different.
- The emphasis on the history and examination varies greatly with age.
- You need to be an entertainer to get the children to cooperate.
- Do not forget the parents. Show your sensitivity, get their consent, explain to them (as well as the child if possible) the test and findings.
- Parents are often right – listen to them.

How to attract a young child's attention

- With an attractive toy, bubbles
- With interesting sounds: rattle, bunch of keys, musical toys, blow raspberries
- Play peek-a-boo

Dealing with a verbal child

Listen to them. Let them speak. Explain to them what you are doing.
Flatter them to win their cooperation: 'I've been told you are a very fast runner. Can you run to that wall as fast as you can and back to me?'.
Set them a challenge: 'I bet you can't open your mouth as wide as mine'.

Dealing with a screaming/frightened child

Do not remove them from their parents.
Allow space and time for them to calm down.
Give them a toy to hold.
Defer the examination if the child is very distressed.

Examining a child

Start by interacting with the child to get his trust and attention. Explain what you're doing; like adults, children do not like to be surprised and frightened.
Demonstrate. Let him play with your equipment: this will rouse his interest and generate cooperation.

Examining a tender area (try and do this last)

Put the child's hand on the area and palpate over his hand. Increase your pressure very slowly. Watch the child's face.

Taking a history from a parent and child

Introduction

Greet the parent and the child (establish who is accompanying the child). Find out the child's preferred name and use that for the history. Introduce yourself to the child to engage their attention.

Age

In years and months, or days and weeks for babies. For premature babies, calculate their corrected age taking into account the weeks of gestation at birth.

Presenting complaint

Define for the complaint:

- onset
- duration
- previous episodes
- treatment
- associated symptoms, systems inquiry

- effects on child's alertness, behaviour, feeding, sleeping
- Impact on family

Signs and symptoms of an ill child:

- growth problems
- loss of appetite
- quiet and withdrawn
- not being herself/himself
- off school/playgroup
- constant crying
- specific symptoms such as diarrhoea and vomiting

Pain history:

- 'Do you think Billy is in pain?'
- Frequency, duration
- Site: ask the child to point to the area
- Characteristics: ask the child if it is sharp like needles, burning, comes and goes, achy
- What does he do when the pain starts: rub the area, scream, lie very still and quiet, roll around on the floor, vomit or feel sick?
- Alleviating and aggravating factors

Past medical history

Include visits to GP, A&E.

Neonatal history

Problems in pregnancy
Maternal complications: blood pressure, gestational diabetes, thyroid disease, drug treatment
Mode of delivery
Term/premature
Postnatal problems

Growth and developmental history

Ask to see the child's record for height, weight and head circumference centiles (The Red Book)
'Do you have any concerns about his weight and height?'
'Has Billy achieved all his developmental milestones so far?'
'Do you have any concerns regarding his development?'

Immunization

'Is Billy up to date with all his vaccinations?' If necessary, ask to see the child's record book, the 'Red Book'. Know the standard vaccination schedule.

Nutrition

For an infant, ask if they are breast fed or bottle fed, volume and frequency of feeds. For an older infant, ask when solids were introduced.

Drug and allergy history

Family history

Depending on the presenting complaint, the family history takes on different emphases.

- Siblings: ages and names and their significant medical histories
- Hereditary diseases
- Consanguinity of parents
- Infectious disease: does anyone in the family have the same symptoms as Billy?
- Be able to draw a family tree to include parents, siblings and step-siblings.

Social history

Home:

- Who lives with the child?
- Parents' marital status and occupation
- Housing
- Financial support
- Do parents smoke?
- Where does the child sleep?

School:

- Attendance?
- Is the child in the appropriate year?
- Any problems mixing with other children? Bullying?
- Any concerns with his capabilities?
- If the child has special needs or learning difficulties, is he statemented*? What is the degree of severity?

*The Statement of Special Educational Needs is a report produced by members of the community paediatric teams stating what support and resources would allow a child to flourish. The child is entitled to this under the 1993 Education Act.

Summary

Summarize the history.

Close the discussion by asking if there are any other problems to discuss. Encourage questions from parents and child. Explain differential diagnosis, plans of investigations.

OSCE scenarios and key features in the history

Child with cough/wheeze

- Sputum/haemoptysis (e.g. older child with cystic fibrosis)
- Fever
- Night time mainly/exercise related dry cough (asthma)
- Allergen contact
- Stridor, saliva pooling, fever (epiglottitis), life-threatening and therefore very unlikely in an OSCE
- Bark-like cough, hoarse voice, afebrile, stridor (croup)
- Failure to thrive (cystic fibrosis)
- Family History (Atopy)
- Environment (smoking)

Child with fever and rash

- Fever or rash first? Time lapse between them
- Rash distribution, spreading? – face/trunk/nappy area
- Appearance of rash: raised, flat, crops, red, discharging, non-blanching (petechial rash of meningitis)
- Itching and scratching
- Headache, vomiting, seizure, fever, photophobia conscious level (meningitis)?
- Contact history: siblings/classmates with rash too?
- Vaccinations: MMR?

Child with fits

- Onset, frequency, duration of fit, witnesses?
- Nature of fits: jerking, absences, limp body, loss of consciousness, tongue biting or incontinence
- Warning signs: dizziness, pallor, aura, angry screaming (breath holding induced?)
- Postictal state: confused, sleepy, normal
- Fever related (febrile convulsions, meningitis)

- Headache and vomiting (raised intracranial pressure?)
- Perinatal problems? Developmental delay?

Child with vomiting

- Onset, frequency, amount and contents of vomitus
- Dehydrated? Wet nappies, urine output, fluid/milk intake
- Projectile, soon after feed (pyloric stenosis, generally around 5 weeks)
- Bile stained (obstruction)
- Blood stained (oesophagitis gastritis)
- Irritablity or abdominal pain? (could be a UTI but exclude intussuception)
- Abdominal pain and diarrhoea (gastroenteritis)
- Pain elsewhere (vomiting due to pain)

Child with diarrhoea

- Onset, frequency
- Dehydrated? Wet nappies, fluid/milk intake
- Abdominal pain, vomiting
- Food related
- Failure to thrive (coeliac disease, cystic fibrosis)
- Soft, pale sticky stool, steatorrhoea (coeliac disease, cystic fibrosis)
- Blood stained (necrotizing enterocolitis, intussuception)

Paediatric cardiac examination

Introduction

Introduce yourself to the child and parents. Establish rapport with the child.

Exposure and position

Ask for the child to be undressed to the waist. Position the child at 45°.

General inspection

Dysmorphic features?
Respiratory distress and tachypnoea?
Colour: blue or pallor?
Sweating?
Count respiratory rate?

Hands

Clubbing, splinter haemorrhages on nails, capillary refill
Pallor on palmar creases
Brachial pulses and femoral pulses, more useful than radial pulses in young
 children. Assess for:

- rate
- volume
- radio (brachial)-femoral delay

TABLE 30.1   Normal pulse rates in children (at rest)

Age	Rate (pulse/min)
<1 year	100–160
2–4 years	90–140
4–10 years	80–140
>10 years	65–100

Eye

Pallor, Jaundice?

Tongue

Central cyanosis?

Carotid pulses

Warn the child first. Check the pulse gently.

Inspection of chest

Scars
Shape and symmetry
JVP

Palpation

Apex beat: use the palm of your hand. Fifth intercostal space, left
 midclavicular line
Heaves and thrills

Auscultation

Praecordium

Use the diaphragm of the stethoscope. Warn the child what you are about to do. Listen over the four valvular areas:

- aortic (right sternal border, second intercostal space)
- pulmonary (left sternal border, second intercostal space)
- tricuspid (left sternal border, fourth intercostal space)
- mitral (apex)

Listen to the heart sounds:

- murmurs: timing, site of maximum intensity, radiation
- loudness: grade out of 6 (1 barely audible, 2 soft, 3 loud with no thrill, 4 loud with thrill, 5 very loud with thrill, 6 audible without stethoscope)

Back

Sit the patient up and listen to the back for:

- crackles in pulmonary oedema (rare)
- radiation of murmurs to back

TABLE 30.2   Differences between innocent and significant murmurs

Innocent	Significant
Midsystolic	Pansystolic, all diastolic
Soft (grades 1–3)	Loud (grades 4–6)
Localized	Radiates throught praecordium
Asymptomatic	Heave, thrill, displaced apex, etc.

Palpate for hepatomegaly

Lie the patient flat at this stage and palpate from the right iliac fossa upwards. Note the liver edge in centimetres below the costal margin.

Ankles and shins

Palpate for peripheral oedema.

Finally

Say you would examine the child's blood pressure (with child/infant cuff). Thank the child and parents. Help the child get dressed.

Likely cases in OSCE*

TABLE 30.3   Likely cases in OSCE

	Timing	Radiation	Other signs
Ventricular septal defect	Pansystolic	All over	Thrill and heave The smaller the VSD, the louder the murmur
Atrial septal defect	Systolic	Pulmonary area	Fixed splitting of second heart sound
Aortic stenosis	Ejection systolic	Neck	Sudden collapse on exertion (on History)
Coartaction of the aorta	Systolic	Back	Radiofemoral delay or absent femoral pulses, hypertension
Persistent ductus arteriosus	Continuous machinery	Back	

Paediatric chest examination

Introduction

Exposure and position

Ask for the child to be undressed to the waist. Sit or position the child at 45° or, for a baby, on his back. In an ill child, use whatever position they are comfortable in.

General inspection

Does the child look ill? Alertness, colour
Obvious dysmorphic features?
Is the child small for his age?
Is the breathing difficult?

● Pursed lip breathing
● Nasal flaring (grunting and headbobbing are unlikely as these are acute signs of respiratory distress)
● Use of accessory muscles

Measure respiratory rate (over 10 s)
Listen for: cough, wheezes, stridor, croup or barking cough
Patches of eczema (atopic with asthma)

*Other OSCEs may involve post-surgical children.

TABLE 30.4   Paediatric respiratory rates

	Normal respiratory rate/min (at rest)	Tachypnoea (rate/min)
Newborn	30–50	>60
Infant	20–30	>50
Toddler	20–30	>40
Children	15–20	>30

Inspect chest

Be seen to inspect closely the anterior and posterior chest walls and under the axillae
Chest deformities:

- pectus excavatum: hollow chest
- pectus carinatum: pigeon chest

Harrison's sulcus (chronic respiratory distress)
Symmetrical chest movement?
Intercostal recession
Scars

Hands

Clubbing, anaemia, cyanosis

Tongue

Central cyanosis

Cervical lymph nodes

Cervical lymphadenopathy can indicate infection or malignancy.

Palpation

Warm your hands first and warn the child. Spread your hands wide on each side of the chest and the thumbs should meet in the midline. Ask the child to breathe in and out through their mouth – demonstrate.

- Chest expansion: your thumbs should spread by 3–5 cm in school-age children. Is the expansion symmetrical?
- Tracheal deviation: be gentle as this can be distressing for the child.

Percussion – anterior chest

Warn the child that you are going to tap on his chest 'like a drum'.

Starting from the apex of the lung, percuss down anteriorly at the upper, middle and lower lung fields and then the midaxillary line. Compare the left and right sides as you descend.

- Hyper-resonance: asthma, pneumothorax (less likely)
- Dullness: consolidation; over liver, which will be elevated if there is collapsed lung above; stony dullness – pleural effusion

Auscultation – anterior chest

Use the bell of an adult stethoscope if a paediatric stethoscope is not available. Warm it up before use. Ask the child to open his mouth and breathe in and out.

Listen to the breath sounds anteriorly at the upper, middle and lower lung fields and then the midaxillary line. Compare the left and right sides. Ask the child to say '99' and listen for vocal fremitus.

Breath sounds:

- vesicular (inspiration followed by expiration without a break – normal)
- bronchial (with a pause in between inspiration and expiration – consolidation)
- increased (consolidation)
- decreased (effusion, pneumothorax)

Added sounds: wheezes, crackles
Vocal fremitus:

- increased (consolidation)
- decreased (effusion, pneumothorax)

Percussion and auscultation – posterior chest

Sit the child forward and repeat percussion and auscultation on the back.

Finally

Say you'd like to perform an ENT exam and check PEFR (if over 6 years old). Thank the child and parent, help the child get dressed.

Most likely OSCE cases

Usually stable patients with chronic diseases, such as asthma and cystic fibrosis.

Paediatric abdominal examination

Introduction

Position and exposure

The ideal position is to lie the child flat on the couch, although they might feel threatened by this. Expose from the nipples to the knees, respecting dignity as appropriate.

General inspection

Is the child small for age?
Dysmorphic features?
Jaundice
Nasogastric tube

Hands

Palmar erythema, anaemia, clubbing, koilonychia

Eyes

Jaundice and anaemia

Mouth

Perioral pigmentation (Peutz–Jeghers syndrome)
Aphthous ulcers. Dry mucous membranes (dehydration)

Inspection of abdomen

Scars
Distension: faecal loading, ascites, intestinal obstruction, obesity
Umbilical hernia
Visible peristalsis
Roll the child to the sides to inspect the flanks fully as well

Palpation

Always ask the child: 'Does your tummy hurt? Point to the area that hurts'. Explain what you are going to do. Demonstrate on a toy if needed. Look at the child's face during palpation.

Bend down or kneel to the child's level. Palpate with your palm, superficially in the four quadrants, then deeply. Elicit:

- tenderness
- guarding
- masses

Liver edge:

- start in the right iliac fossa, moving up, asking the child to breathe in as you palpate
- can be felt 1–2 cm below the right costal margin

Spleen:

- start in the left iliac fossa, moving up (right iliac fossa in younger children)
- repeat with the child rolled to the right
- the spleen is just palpable in an infant but not in an older child

Kidneys:

- bimanual approach: with your left hand under the flanks and right hand anteriorly, try to ballot the kidneys between both hands
- are they enlarged? Is one absent?

TABLE 30.5   Characteristics of the abdominal organs in children (note differences between left kidney and spleen, which can be easily confused)

Liver	Kidney	Spleen
Palpable edge normally	Usually not palpable	Palpable in infants usually Not palpable in older children
Unable to get above, but upper border can be percussed	Able to get above	Unable to get above (even if enlarged)
–	Ballotable bimanually	Not ballotable
–	No notching	Notch present
Enlarges towards the right iliac fossa	–	Enlarges downwards towards the left iliac fossa in infants, but diagonally towards the right iliac fossa in older children

Percussion

Warn the child that you are about to 'tap on their tummy like a drum'.
Percuss over the four quadrants.
Percuss out to the upper and lower borders of the liver.

Percuss the subrapubic area for a distended bladder.

For a distended abdomen, demonstrate shifting dullness and fluid thrill for ascites.

- Shifting dullness: starting from the umbilicus, percuss towards the flank and mark the site at which it becomes dull. Turn the child towards you and percuss again. The transition to dullness will have moved towards the midline in the presence of peritoneal fluid.
- Fluid thrill: place the side of your right hand on the left side of the abdomen, facing the child. Gently flick the opposite side of the abdomen and feel for the transmission of a thrill.

Auscultate

Bowel sounds

Finally

Say you'd like to examine the:

- genitalia
- inguinal region for herniae
- anal area
- rectal area (rarely such as cases of severe constipation, or encopresis)

Thank the child and parents and help the child get dressed.

Likely OSCE cases

Many patients with organomegaly or gastrointestinal disorders will be well enough to be examined.

- Hepatomegaly, splenomegaly and kidney mass
- Colostomies, ileostomies
- Chronic liver/renal diseases
- Constipation and faecal loading
- Crohn's disease, ulcerative colitis
- Cystic fibrosis with liver involvement

Paediatric neurological examination

In an older child who follows commands, the neurological exam can be performed as in an adult. For infants and toddlers, the bulk of the exam involves observation of their play and interaction. Demonstrate what you want them to do through play. Make it fun and enjoyable.

Introduction

Introduce yourself to the child and parents. Establish rapport with the child.

Brief history

Reduced movement *in utero*
Premature birth
Birth trauma
Emergency caesarean section
Perinatal asphyxiation
Low Apgar score
Family History

General observation

Alertness, posture
Dysmorphic features
Walking aids/wheelchair
Speech and language: are they vocalizing/talking as appropriate for their age?
Social interaction (NEVER assume that a physically handicapped child is mentally handicapped)

Limp

Ask the child to walk, run, jump and skip. Also test heel–toe walking. For young children, tempt them with a toy to assess their mobility.

- Is the child's gross motor function appropriate for their age?
- Is there an abnormal limp, hemiplegia, ataxia, waddling, muscular dystrophy, antalgic limp?

Motor system

Ideally, the motor exam should be done in order of upper limb followed by lower limb. In reality, you might do the same test in both upper and lower limb for convenience or be opportunistic in an uncooperative child and do it in a random order.

Inspection

Look at all four limbs for: muscle wasting, abnormal posture and contractures.

Tone

Do not forget to ask about pain first. Be gentle.

- Holding the hand, flex and extend the elbow.
- Sit the child down or lie them down. Roll the knees side to side – the feet should flop loosely.
- Pick the knee up and let it drop on the bed – the heel should remain on the bed.

Power

For young children, watch what they can do with their hands and feet to assess power. Ask them to:

- pick a toy up from the ground
- throw a ball back to you
- pull a toy from your grasp
- kick a ball.

In older children, assess formally. Make it fun and challenge them: 'I bet you are not as strong as I am'.

Upper limb:
- shoulder abduction and adduction
- elbow flexion and extension
- wrist flexion

Lower limb:
- hip flexion and extension
- knee flexion and extension
- ankle plantarflexion and dorsiflexion

Reflexes

Sit the child down or lie them down. Explain you are trying to see how bouncy their arms and legs are.

Use a paediatric tendon hammer. For children less than 12 months old, consider tapping over the joints with your fingers. Check the following reflexes:

- biceps
- triceps
- knee
- ankle

Check for clonus. Sharply dorsiflex the ankle. More than three beats of clonus is pathological.

Coordination

For young children, this is done by observation for incoordination.

For older children, perform finger-to-nose test and demonstrate dysdiodochokinesis. Ask them to walk heel to toe like on a tightrope.

Perform the heel–shin test by asking the child to rub their heels on the contralateral shin.

Sensation

Sensation is usually unreliable in a young child. For older children, test the following modalities along the upper and lower limb dermatomes (see Chapters 16 and 20 on adult neurology for details):

- Light touch
- Proprioception
- Vibration sense

Cranial nerves

If the child is old enough, this can be done like an adult's examination.

Likely OSCE cases

Cerebral palsy
Duchenne/Becker muscular dystrophy

Part 6

Practical skills

31 Basic life support and advanced life support

It is the bare minimum of any healthcare professional to be expected to perform adequate Basic Life Support (BLS). Advanced Life Support is carried out by a dedicated team which includes the medical team, anaesthetist and Hospital Resuscitation Officers.

Basic life support (BLS)

Scenario

You are walking through a corridor in your hospital and find a person lying unconscious on the floor.

- Assess for danger – is there a reason why this person is on the floor, e.g. any live wires and water?
- Try to rouse them – 'shake and shout'.
- If responsive, put into recovery position.
- If no response, call for help.

ABC

A Airway

- Head tilt, chin lift (as if the person were 'sniffing the morning air') (Figure 31.1).
- If you suspect a cervical spine injury, perform a jaw thrust.

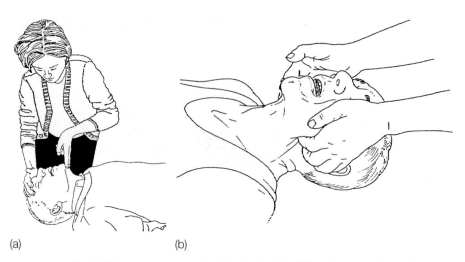

(a)   (b)

FIGURE 31.1 Establishing an airway. (a) Head tilt. (b) Chin lift. (Copyright European Resuscitation Council, reproduced with permission.)©

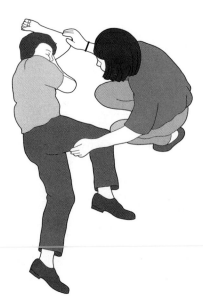

FIGURE 31.2 The recovery position. (Copyright European Resuscitation Council; reproduced with permission.)©

- Check the mouth for foreign objects: well-fitting dentures should stay in as they help keep the airway intact.
- Consider a finger sweep.

B Breathing

- Assess by placing your face over the mouth and looking down at the chest wall for movement, listening for breath sounds and feeling for breath on your cheek – *look, listen and feel*. Do this for 10 seconds.
- If they are breathing, they will have a pulse and you can place them in the recovery position (Figure 31.2).
- If they are not breathing, and you have ensured that the airway is clear (to the best of your ability), leave the patient (if you are alone) and put out a *crash call*.
- Know the number for the hospital at which your examination is being held.
- Repeat the call twice to make sure the team arrive at the correct location: 'Cardiac arrest, corridor, blue zone, level 2. Cardiac arrest, corridor, blue zone, level 2.'
- If there is another health professional, say 'Please put out a cardiac arrest call, get a bag-valve mask and return to let me know you've done that'.

C Circulation

- Feel for the carotid for 10 seconds; this should be done whilst you are looking, listening and feeling for breath sounds.
- If there is a pulse, continue to rescue breath until help arrives.
- If there is no pulse, your priority is to summon help. If this is a 'shockable' rhythm you need the defibrillator *immediately*.
- If you are alone, leave the patient and call the crash team, before returning to perform CPR.

Commence CPR

Begin with two rescue breaths, preferably with a bag-valve mask connected to oxygen (Figure 31.3) but by mouth-to-mouth if necessary. After each breath, check if you were successful by watching the chest fall.

If after five attempts, you are not successful, move on to chest compressions.* Chest compressions should be performed at a rate of 100 per

---

*Chest compressions will move air in and out of the lungs, so the patient will have some degree of oxygenation, as long as there is not a total occlusion of the upper airway.

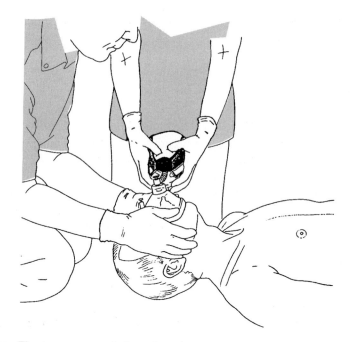

FIGURE 31.3 The two-person technique for using a bag-valve-mask. (Copyright European Resuscitation Council; reproduced with permission.)©

minute, with the heel of your palm, two finger breadths above the sternal notch. In an adult, you should aim for 3–4 cm depth of compression.

Do this at a rate of 15 compressions to two breaths. If you are aided, ask the health professional to start by doing the breathing whilst you compress and swap when you feel you are tiring.

After each minute (approximately three cycles), stop and reassess the patient.

Continue till help arrives or you are exhausted. Deciding when continuation is futile is best left to a more experienced doctor.

During these cycles of BLS, you may have access to airway adjuncts.

- Oropharyngeal (Guedel): estimate the size needed by placing the airway against the face and choosing that which best represents the vertical distance between the patient's incisors and the angle of the jaw. Start by pushing gently in with the tip pointing towards the roof of the mouth, and then twist through 180° so that it holds the tongue in place.
- Nasopharyngeal: measure by checking that the diameter is roughly the same as the patient's little finger. Push with the bevel end first vertically along the floor of the nose.

The crash team should now arrive. With you being the first at the scene and the only doctor there, you are in charge…

Advanced life support (ALS)

This must always be preceded by basic life support (see above).

Reassess your patient – are they still apnoeic and pulseless?

Expose the chest and get the electrode pads on: right apex – just below right clavicle; left – by cardiac apex.

Be sure to remove any patches (GTN, nicotine, as these are potentially explosive) and place the pads at least 15 cm away from any pacemaker.

Get the monitor on and ask the person performing compressions to stop for a moment.

You will now see one of four possible outputs:

A. Pulseless ventricular tachycardia (pulseless VT)

B. Ventricular fibrillation (VF)

C. Pulseless electrical activity (PEA): normal ECG morphology, accompanied by no cardiac output

D. Asystole: the absence of any morphology – a 'flatline'

Make a note to check that you:

- are reading from LEAD II
- have the gain set to +1 (move it up if you suspect asystolic readout is false – it will remain flat no matter how high you set it)
- have the pads on and positioned correctly.

Rhythms A and B are 'shockable'; that is, they may respond to defibrillation with DC current. Rhythms C and D are not.

Shockable rhythms

- Clear everyone away from the patient and make sure the oxygen is not attached to any tube that might be in situ.
- Announce and check: 'Clear top, clear middle, clear bottom, clear self, oxygen away'.
- Charge to 200 J: 'Charging'.
- Perform another visual sweep to make sure everyone is clear.
- 'Patient is in VF/pulseless VT, delivering shock, stand clear.'
- Deliver shock.
- If no rhythm change, repeat process.

- If there is still no rhythm change, ask that charge is set to 360 J, then deliver shock as above.

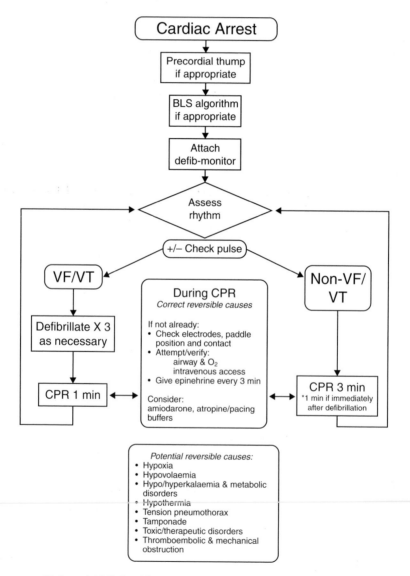

FIGURE 31.4 Universal ALS algorithm.

After the third cycle, perform CPR for one minute. During this minute, you and the team need to assess:

A. Airway adjunct: if you manage to get an endotracheal tube (ETT) you can perform asynchronous CPR, that is, continuous compressions and breathing
B. Ventilations should be accompanied by 100% O_2, ABGs
C. Inotropic support: 1 mg adrenaline (10 ml of 1 in 10,000); 300 mg amiodarone (given for VF/pulseless VT that has not responded to defibrillation, i.e. it is 'refractory')
D. Pupils (has patient stroked/overdosed?), BMs
E. Exposure: any signs of bleeding, particularly intra-abdominally?

Perform another three cycles, staying at 360 J from now on. Continue until patient is revived or resuscitation is deemed futile by an experienced doctor.

Non-shockable rhythms

- Perform three minutes CPR.
- Reassess the patient.
- Assess as above but give: 1 mg adrenaline (10 ml of 1 in 10,000); 3 mg atropine – ONCE ONLY in asystole or in PEA if heart rate <60.
- If no response, perform another three minutes CPR.

TABLE 31.1   The 4 Hs and the 4 Ts

Problem	Signs	Management
Hypovolaemia	Active bleeding, dry	Rapid fluids, O neg. blood
Hypothermia	Feels cold, low core temperature	Warm fluids
Hypoxia	Universal, ABGs	100% O_2
Hyperkalaemia, hypocalcaemia, acidaemia	Bloods, ECG, ABGs	Calcium carbonate for ↑K^+ and ↓Ca^{2+} Sodium bicarbonate for acidosis
Tension pneumothorax	Penetrating injury, no breath sounds, displaced trachea	Needle thoracocentesis
Tamponade	↑JVP, history chest trauma	Pericardiocentesis
Thromboembolism (i.e. PE)	History of immobility, pelvic surgery, pregnancy, etc.	Thrombolysis
Toxic/therapeutic	History	Supportive, specific antidotes if known agent

Reversible causes

As team leader, it is up to you to consider whether there is a definite reversible cause for this cardiac arrest. These are the 4 Hs and the 4 Ts (Table 31.1).

If the patient develops a cardiac output

A + B Airway and breathing

Oxygenate and ventilate if necessary
Check placement of ETT
CXR

C Circulation

Cardiac monitor
BP

D + E Disability and exposure

Glasgow Coma Score and log roll

F Family

Offer to speak to them and explain what has happened.

G Gratitude

Thank the team for their swift arrival and assistance.

32 Prescribing

This is a common source of panic ... but simple enough with practice and a few pointers. Regardless of the situation you are presented with, you can be awarded about a third of the available marks in an OSCE for simply filling in the patient details.

Remember

- Name – forename and surname
- Hospital and ward (usually A&E)
- Consultant – use your imagination. Or Dr Smith.
- HO's name and bleep – that's you!
- Unit number
- DOB
- Age/sex
- Drug sensitivity – No Known Drug Allergies

Some typical cases

- You are a PRHO on call in A&E. You see Mr Jonathan Brent, who presents with 'crushing' central chest pain. Mr Brent's ECG shows widespread ST elevation and inverted T waves. He has been taking verapamil 240 mg tds for hypertension and develops urticaria when taking penicillin. His Unit No. is 156823 and his DOB is 4/12/1943.
- You are a PRHO on call in A&E. You see Mr Jack Spade, who presents with

breathlessness and wheezing and is coughing up pink, frothy sputum. He has had an MI in the last year and is on atenolol 50 mg od and simvastatin 40 mg od. On examination he is tachycardic and tachypnoeic. Mr Spade has no known drug allergies. His Unit No. is 548732 and his DOB is 20/04/1952.

- You are a PRHO on call in A&E. A secretary, Joanne Morris, is admitted with acute breathlessness. She has had a three-day history of a cough productive of green sputum and a history of asthma since childhood. She regularly takes a Becloforte inhaler twice daily, salbutamol inhaler and currently diazepam 5 mg om for trouble sleeping. On examination she is tachycardic and tachypnoeic with a widespread expiratory wheeze and reduced air entry bilaterally. She has no known drug allergies. Her Unit No. is 024835 and her DOB is 10/08/1980.

- You are a PRHO on call in A&E. You see Mr Andrew Tang, who presents with N+V and dyspepsia. He looks pale and sweaty and has vomited up what looks like coffee grounds. He has a known history of angina and is currently taking glyceryl trinitrate (GTN) two puffs bd, lansoprazole 30 mg od, aspirin 75 mg od. His Unit No. is 205486 and his DOB is 20/07/1969.

- You are the PRHO for Dr Johnson's team. You are called to see Ellie Knight, a dental student, who was treated for a chest infection by her GP. She now (in addition to her chest symptoms) is complaining of a swollen tongue and you are sure her face looks swollen. She is taking augmentin 625 mg tds (six days left) and has no known drug allergies. Her Unit No. is 197826 and her DOB is 22/10/80.

- You are the PRHO in A&E. You are asked to write up Mr John Blair's drug chart. He presents with an acutely hot, tender, swollen, painful right first metatarsophalangeal joint. Joint aspirate microscopy has revealed negatively birefringent crystals. He has a history of a stomach ulcer when he was younger. He is on bendrofluazide 2.5 mg om for high blood pressure. His Unit No. is 9289292 and his DOB is 10/02/48.

- You are the PRHO in orthopaedics. One of your patients admitted four days ago, Mr Peter Dent (Unit No. 1963666, DOB 31/10/45), is being discharged today, following a left knee arthroscopy and medial meniscectomy three days ago (diagnosis: osteoarthritis of left knee). The procedure was more painful than expected and your consultant has asked that the patient goes home with three days of Sevredol (oral morphine) to be taken as required up to four times a day whilst he gets back on his feet. Otherwise he is healthy and had an uneventful stay. He is also taking aspirin 75 mg in the mornings and simvastatin 40 mg in the evenings. As well as Sevredol PRN, he has been taking regular paracetamol and dihydrocodeine in hospital. He has a red wristband with penicillin written on it. His address and GP details have been filled out by the ward clerk. Please complete his discharge summary and prescription. He is to be seen in Mr Allen's clinic in two weeks.

A few things to remember…

- For each drug: generic name, dose, route (iv, neb, po, etc.), start date, when to give and **signature**.
- For 'When to give', the timing rarely matters in finals, as long as it's obvious that it's either od/bd/tds, etc. For O_2, a vertical arrow through all time boxes indicates continuous deliverance.
- Some drugs need to be stopped (sedatives in respiratory distress, calcium channel inhibitors in an MI). If so, write it up and then cross it out.
- For GTN or asthma inhaler, T = puff, TT = 2 puffs.
- Discharge summaries are potentially fair game on prescription stations. Remember to include anything the patient was taking in hospital. Most hospitals prescribe for up to two weeks. Some drugs, such as opiates or antibiotics, will be prescribed for less.

Bearing these points in mind, make copies of the prescription chart in Figure 32.1 and practise the above vignettes under examination conditions.

Points to bear in mind for the above vignettes*

Treatment of myocardial infarct

Remember 'Moan':

- **M**orphine 5–10 mg IV/IM and metoclopramide 10 mg IM
- **O**$_2$ (60%)
- **A**spirin 300 mg po
- **N**itrate (GTN) sublingual (consider infusion).

Stop verapamil; calcium antagonists are contraindicated (cardiac conduction defects)
Note penicillin allergy (even though it may not be immediately relevant)
Consider adding *regular*: aspirin, simvastatin, β-blocker, ACE inhibitor

Treatment of pulmonary oedema

- Morphine 2.5–10 mg and metoclopramide 10 mg

*Guidelines and medications will change, and vary between hospitals. Prescribe safely and you will pass.

continued on p 245 …

St Toby's Hospital
NHS Trust

Drug Prescription

Student Name

Student Number

WARD		
UNIT No.		
SURNAME		
FIRST NAME		
DATE OF BIRTH		
CONSULTANT		
HOUSE OFFICER		Bleep No.
Date of Admission		

DETAILS OF PREVIOUS/ADMISSION MEDICATION – TO BE COMPLETED BY DOCTER

DRUG	DOSE	DIRECTIONS	DURATION OF TREATMENT

DRUGS NOT ADMINISTERED

DATE	TIME	DRUG	NURSE'S SIGNATURE	REASON

Name:

WEIGHT: HEIGHT:

Use approved names. NO ABBREVIATIONS.
Any changes in drug therapy must be ordered by a new prescription. DO NOT ALTER EXISTING INSTRUCTIONS.
Discontinue a drug by drawing a line through it.

DRUG ALLERGIES

REGULAR PRESCRIPTIONS

DATE AND MONTH →			
TICK TIMES OR ENTER VARIABLE DOSE →			

DRUG (APPROVED NAME)				7
Dose	Route	Start Date	Valid Period	9
				13
		Pharmacy		18
				22
Additional Information				

DRUG (APPROVED NAME)				7
Dose	Route	Start Date	Valid Period	9
				13
Signature		Pharmacy		18
				22
Additional Information				

DRUG (APPROVED NAME)				7
Dose	Route	Start Date	Valid Period	9
				13
Signature		Pharmacy		18
				22
Additional Information				

DRUG (APPROVED NAME)				7
Dose	Route	Start Date	Valid Period	9
				13
Signature		Pharmacy		18
				22
Additional Information				

DRUG (APPROVED NAME)				7
Dose	Route	Start Date	Valid Period	9
				13
Signature		Pharmacy		18
				22
Additional Information				

DRUG (APPROVED NAME)				7
Dose	Route	Start Date	Valid Period	9
				13
Signature		Pharmacy		18
				22
Additional Information				

AS REQUIRED PRESCRIPTIONS

DRUG (APPROVED NAME)				Date															
Dose	Route	Start Date	Valid Period	Time															
Signature		Max. Freq.	Pharmacy	Dose															
Additional Information				Given by															
DRUG (APPROVED NAME)				Date															
Dose	Route	Start Date	Valid Period	Time															
Signature		Max. Freq.	Pharmacy	Dose															
Additional Information				Given by															
DRUG (APPROVED NAME)				Date															
Dose	Route	Start Date	Valid Period	Time															
Signature		Max. Freq.	Pharmacy	Dose															
Additional Information				Given by															
DRUG (APPROVED NAME)				Date															
Dose	Route	Start Date	Valid Period	Time															
Signature		Max. Freq.	Pharmacy	Dose															
Additional Information				Given by															
DRUG (APPROVED NAME)				Date															
Dose	Route	Start Date	Valid Period	Time															
Signature		Max. Freq.	Pharmacy	Dose															
Additional Information				Given by															
DRUG (APPROVED NAME)				Date															
Dose	Route	Start Date	Valid Period	Time															
Signature		Max. Freq.	Pharmacy	Dose															
Additional Information				Given by															
DRUG (APPROVED NAME)				Date															
Dose	Route	Start Date	Valid Period	Time															
Signature		Max. Freq.	Pharmacy	Dose															
Additional Information				Given by															

ONCE ONLY AND PREMEDICATION DRUGS

DATE	DRUG	DOSE	TIME	ROUTE	SIGNATURE	Time given	Given by	PHARMACY

FIGURE 32.1   Sample of a drug prescription chart.

- Note that patient came in on certain drugs. Note also the patient's blood pressure, if this is included; you may need to stop any drugs with a negative inotropic effect.
- Frusemide 40 mg po (consider IV); can be increased to 80 mg
- O_2 (60%)

Treatment of asthma

Remember 'O Shit!':

- O_2
- Salbutamol 5 mg nebs (2–4 hourly) regular or PRN or both

- **H**ydrocortisone 100–200 mg IV/prednisolone 40 mg od; continue the regular inhaled steroid
- **I**pratropium 250 μg nebs qds
- **T**heophylline? (get SHO to think about this)

Consider antibiotics if you suspect a chest infection; paracetamol.

Stop any sedatives.

Anaphylaxis

This is a medical emergency. Senior help should be summoned. In terms of prescription, the likeliest culprit is the augmentin, which needs to be replaced with another antibiotic. However, the patient needs to be on high-flow oxygen by mask and 0.5–1 mg of adrenaline IM should be administered ASAP. Chlorpheniramine 10–20 mg should be administered as a slow IV injection, along with IV hydrocortisone (100–300 mg).* Nebulized inhalers are a good idea.

Discharging a patient/prescribing a controlled drug

Fill out the patient's details (handwritten – a sticky label will not do), admission date, procedure and date, diagnosis, and your details. Prescribe any drugs the patient was taking in hospital which you wish to continue, and for how long. Remember that for controlled drugs the total amount to take home must be written in words and numbers. Paracetamol for postoperative analgesia is usually 1 g qds and dihydrocodeine (aka DF118) 30 mg qds. These are not 'controlled' and may be prescribed for two weeks.

Patient with suspected peptic ulcer/upper GI bleed

Regular: oxygen, fluids, PPI (lansoprazole or omeprazole infusion). Stop the NSAID if you suspect a PU.
PRN: paracetamol, may need opiate analgesia. May need blood (in fluids section).

Patient with gout

Regular: paracetamol. Indomethacin (3/7 max) or colchicine; this is a strong NSAID so prescribe with a proton pump inhibitor. Fluids, for 24 hours. Allopurinol (if not already on it); this comes later as may worsen attack initially.
PRN: oxygen, codeine phosphate. Aspirin and thiazide diuretics are contraindicated. If in heart failure, use ACE inhibitor instead.

*Jones O. Managing a suspected adverse drug reaction, Student BMJ 2001;9:274-5.

33

Confirmation of death

The typical scenario in this station is you playing the on-call House Officer asked to confirm the death of a patient on a ward (one you did not know yourself) at 2 am. Note that although you will usually be confirming that a mannequin is dead in this station, you will be marked on how sensitive you are, so do take this seriously. The examiner will tell you what your findings are at each point.

1. Speak to Sister/Staff Nurse in charge. Introduce yourself, explain why you're there and ask for a brief history of the patient, including when the patient was last seen alive and by whom.
2. Consider and enquire about the factors shown in the box, which may present to the unwary as a dead patient but are reversible.

Testing for death. Exclude before you SHINE your torch

Sedative drugs: has the patient taken any?
Hypothermia: you cannot exclude death below 35°C; if the temperature is below this you must warm the patient and reassess
Intoxication: depressants and relaxants
Neuromuscular blocking drugs: said relaxants
Electrolyte/Acid balance abnormality – and hypoglycaemia

---

3. Ask for the notes, drug chart and observations for the patient, as well as an ophthalmoscope.
4. Ask the nurse if he or she would accompany you to the patient's bedside.
5. Check the patient's name against the notes and on his or her name tag (and, if applicable, your briefing).

6. Attempt to rouse the patient:
   - Say the patient's name – first gently, then in a *loud* and *clear* voice.
   - First gently then vigorously shake shoulders.
   - Exert pressure on a nail bed and if this does not work...
   - Try a sternal rub; this is a very sensitive test, i.e. very painful.
   - Indicate that you could try a corneal response, if the examiner thinks it necessary.
7. Is the patient breathing?
   - Observe from the bedside for respiratory movements.
   - *Look, listen and feel* over the mouth, i.e. look down the patient's chest for movement, whilst listening for breath sounds and half expecting to feel the patient's breath on your cheek (some people check the carotid pulse at the same time).
   - Auscultate over the lungs: 'I would normally do this for *one minute*, would you like me to do so?'.
8. Feel for pulses on *both* sides.*
   - Carotid: do one at a time here; if patient is not dead, you are theoretically in danger of inducing cerebral ischaemia
   - Radial
   - Femoral
9. Auscultate for heart sounds in each cardiac area with diaphragm: 'I would normally do this for *one minute*, would you like me to do so?'.
10. Does the patient have a pacemaker? State you are looking for one.
11. Ask for the ophthalmoscope and make a decent pretence of performing fundoscopy if you do have a mannequin.
    - Are the pupils fixed and dilated?
    - Look at the retinae: indicate you are looking for 'railroading' of the veins.[†]

Is the patient dead?

Do *all* of the above tests support a diagnosis of death? If not, you would have to assess the need for resuscitation. However, if the station is 'Confirmation of death', the examiner will not turn it into a resuscitation station.

---

*If carotid pulse is palpable, systolic BP is at least 60–70 mmHg; if carotid and femoral pulses are palpable, systolic BP is 70–80 mmHg; and if the radial pulse is also palpable, the systolic BP is >80 mmHg (Deakin and Low, BMJ 321; 2000). Hence if there are no palpable pulses, you know the systolic BP is under 60 mmHg.

[†]This is the description of the appearance of veins containing stationary blood.

12. Record your findings in the notes. A typical example is set out below.

> 12/04/04 – Medical On-call PRHO 0200
>
> Asked to confirm death of patient.
>
> Patient last seen alive at 0000 by ward staff. Was not in any distress.
>
> O/E – Apnoeic, pulseless, no heart sounds. No pacemaker detected.
>
> Pupils fixed and dilated, railroading visible on fundoscopy.
>
> Confirmation of death at 0200 on 12th April 2004.
>
> May he rest in peace.
>
> *John Brown*
>
> John Brown PRHO (Blp 666)

13. State that you will assess whether or not to refer to the Coroner.
14. State that a death certificate needs to be filled out by this patient's regular doctor.
15. State that the GP and next of kin need to be informed, and offer to do so.

34

Interpret and record a 12-lead ECG

Interpret a 12-lead ECG

This will inevitably follow the recording of an ECG. In reality a nurse, who will hand you the printout to interpret, would do the recording. Combining a set of straightforward principles is the key to interpretation of an ECG.

The patient will be known to you, as you will have recorded the ECG yourself. The examiner will tell you that the patient, who is often a young student, is actually a middle-aged man who is experiencing chest pain. They will then hand you an ECG and ask you to interpret it for them.

Morphology of the ECG (Figure 34.1)

P wave: this represents atrial depolarization
QRS complex: ventricular depolarization
T wave: ventricular *re*polarization

The paper speed is normally 25 mm/s, such that each small square represents 0.04 s and each large square represents 0.20 s.

The **PR interval** is the period from the start of the P wave to the start of the QRS complex, normally <5 small squares (<0.20 s). Prolongation represents *first-degree heart block.*

The **QRS duration** is the period from the start to the end of the complex, regardless of which direction the initial deflection is, normally <3 small squares (<0.12 s). Prolongation represents *bundle branch block (BBB).*

The **ST interval** is the period between the end of the QRS complex and the start of the T wave. Usually isoelectric, significant elevation or depression represents myocardial tissue damage, i.e. *MI or ischaemia.*

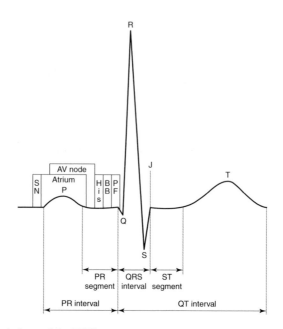

FIGURE 34.1   Morphology of the ECG.

The **QT interval** is the period between the start of the QRS complex and the *end* of the T wave. The corrected QT interval (QT$_c$) is the result of dividing the QT interval by the root of the R-R interval; the ECG machine will do this for you! It is normally <0.44 s. Prolongation is usually drug related and carries a high risk of *ventricular arrhythmias.*

Notes on Q waves

Q waves are normal in aVR, III and V1, due to their position. Pathological Q waves are >0.04 s (one small square) and have a depth of quarter of the R wave of the same lead.

Notes on the QRS complex

If the first deflection of the complex is a *negative* one, this is a *Q wave.*
If the first deflection of the complex is a *positive* one, this is an *R wave,* regardless of whether or not it is preceded by a negative deflection.
Any negative deflection following a positive one is an *S wave.*
A second positive wave is an *R' wave.*
    Bundle branch block (Figure 34.2):

(a)

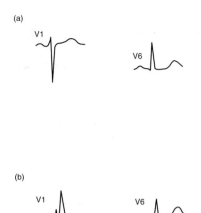

(b)

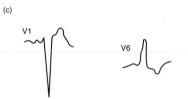

(c)

FIGURE 34.2 Mechanism of ECG appearance of right bundle branch block (RBBB) and left bundle branch block (LBBB). (a) Septal activation from both bundle branches but primarily from the left. (b) RBBB. (c) LBBB.

- left (LBBB): wide Q wave or a small R wave followed by wide S wave in V1. M-shaped complex in V6 (RSR' pattern)
- right (RBBB): M (RSR') or a Q wave followed by a large R wave in V1.

Notes on QRS axis (Figure 34.3)

The wave of depolarization has a direction as well as a magnitude.

The mean frontal QRS vector can be calculated by knowing which leads represent which direction. Using leads I ($0°$) and aVF ($+90°$), the axis can be calculated as being within one of the four quadrants.

- Lead I +ve and aVF +ve: normal axis
- Lead I +ve and aVF −ve:
  - lead II +ve: normal axis
  - lead II −ve: left axis deviation

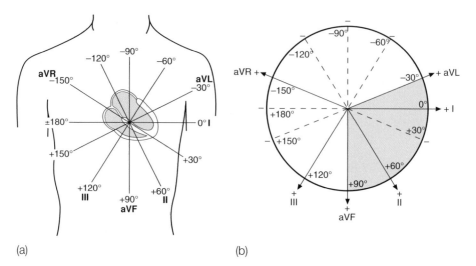

(a)   (b)

FIGURE 34.3   Calculating the axis. A QRS vector directed towards lead I is arbitrarily defined as 0°. Positive axes are directed towards aVL and aVF, and negative axes are directed leftwards towards aVL. Abnormal axes fall outside the -30° (left axis deviation) to 90° (right axis deviation) range.

- Lead I −ve and aVF +ve: right axis deviation
- Lead I −ve and aVF -ve: northwest territory

Notes on ST segment (Figure 34.4)

This segment is usually isoelectric, i.e. it should be flat with no magnitude. Elevation or depression of more than 1 mm is significant in leads I, II, III, aVR, aVL and aVF. In the chest leads, elevation or depression of more than 2 mm is significant.

Significant ST elevation accompanied by chest pain is very suggestive for an acute myocardial infarct.

Notes on T wave (Figure 34.5)

Inverted (negatively deflected) T waves are normal variants in aVR and V1 and are not pathognomonic in leads III and V2. Everywhere else, inverted T waves are abnormal.

When accompanied by pain, this often indicates a subendocardial MI. With no pain, they are more probably indicative of an old MI.

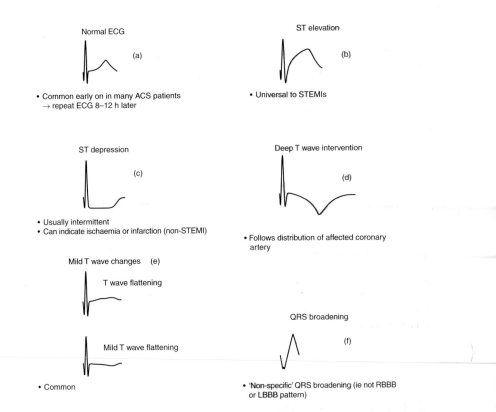

Normal ECG
(a)
- Common early on in many ACS patients
  → repeat ECG 8–12 h later

ST elevation
(b)
- Universal to STEMIs

ST depression
(c)
- Usually intermittent
- Can indicate ischaemia or infarction (non-STEMI)

Deep T wave intervention
(d)
- Follows distribution of affected coronary artery

Mild T wave changes   (e)
T wave flattening

Mild T wave flattening
- Common

QRS broadening
(f)
- 'Non-specific' QRS broadening (ie not RBBB or LBBB pattern)

FIGURE 34.4   ECG changes in acute coronary syndromes (ACS). LAD, left anterior descending coronary artery; LBBB, left bundle branch block; RBBB, right bundle branch block; STEMI, ST segment elevation myocardial infarction.

The readout

Now, use your knowledge of the ECG and of cardiology to go through a readout systematically…

1. Name, DOB, date and time.
2. Calibration (check paper speed).
3. Rate: calculated by dividing the R-R interval (in large squares) into 300, such that a gap of two squares represents 300/2 = 150 bpm, 3 = 100 bpm, 4 = 75 bpm, etc.
4. Rhythm and PR interval: sinus rhythm is by definition when each QRS complex is preceded by a P wave, at a regular interval. Measuring the interval will demonstrate if the patient is in heart block.

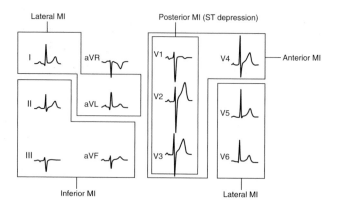

FIGURE 34.5 Basic pattern of ECG changes in myocardial infarction (MI).

5. QRS duration and axis.
6. Pathological Q waves?
7. ST segment changes?
8. T wave inversion?

Combining 6, 7 and 8 can help localize ischaemic or infarctive events (Figure 34.5).

I + aVL, V5 + V6: lateral wall left ventricle
II, III, aVF: inferior wall left ventricle
V1 + V2: right ventricle and interventricular septum
V3 + V4: anterior wall left ventricle

Stations

Atrial fibrillation (Figure 34.6a)

Irregular QRS complexes
Chaotic atrial activity
Best demonstrated in V1

Atrial flutter (Figure 34.6b)

Fast regular activity at 250–300 bpm
Often every other wave gets conducted from the AV node; rate of 125–150 bpm
'Sawtooth' pattern in V1

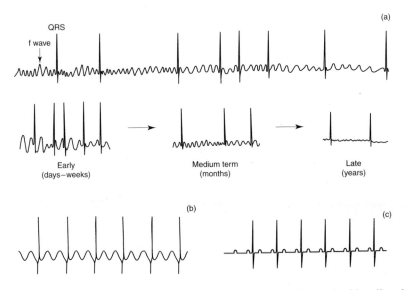

FIGURE 34.6 (a) Atrial fibrillation (AF). The irregular, completely disorganized baseline shows fibrillatory (f) waves and an irregular QRS response. In late AF, f waves are very fine and the baseline may appear almost flat. (b) Atrial flutter. The irregular 'saw-tooth' baseline is best seen in the inferior leads (II, III, aVF) and the heart rate is often a ratio of 300 (i.e. 150, 100 or 75 bpm).

Sinus tachycardia (Figure 34.7)

Broad complex tachycardia when *ventricular*
Narrow complex when *supraventricular*
>100 bpm

Ventricular fibrillation (Figure 34.8)

Broad irregular QRS complexes
Indicates need for immediate defibrillation

Sinus bradycardia (Figure 34.9)

<50 bpm

Heart block

First degree (Figure 34.10a):

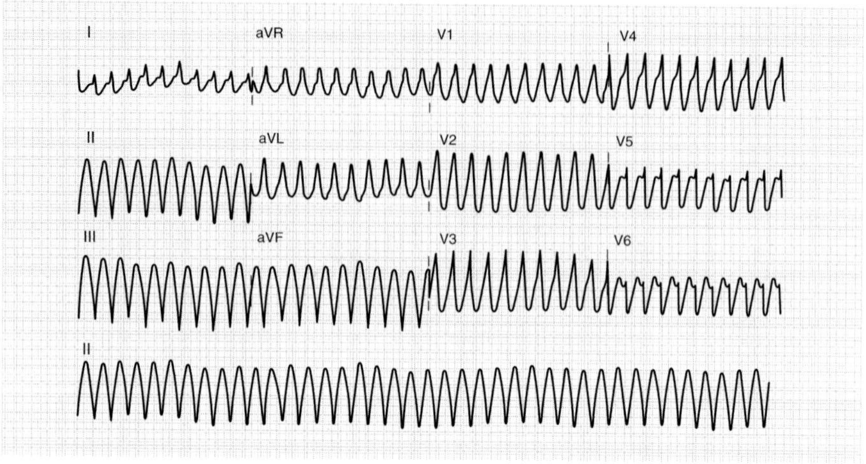

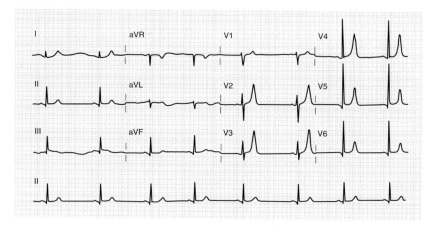

FIGURE 34.7 Sustained monomorphic ventricular tachycardia (VT). This ECG shows a broad complex tachycardia, identified as VT by broad QRS complexes.

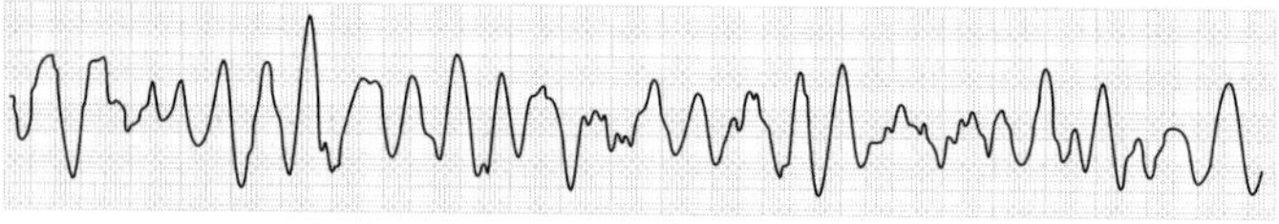

FIGURE 34.8 Ventricular fibrillation (VF).

FIGURE 34.9 Sinus bradycardia. Prominent sinus arrhythmia (irregularity of the PR interval) suggests that the cause of the bradycardia may be a prominent vagal reflex.

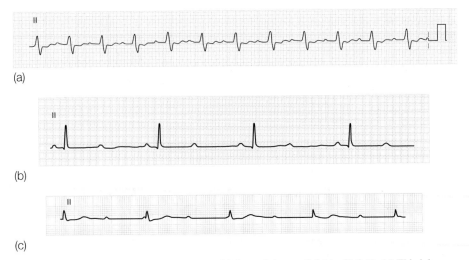

(a)

(b)

(c)

FIGURE 34.10. Heart block. (a) First degree. (b) Second degree (Mobitz II, 2:1). (c) Third degree.

- ↑ PR interval (>0.20 s)
- No symptoms, no treatment required
- Can lead to syncope if accompanied by LBBB or RBBB

Second degree (Figure 34.10b):

- Not all P waves are followed by a QRS complex
- Mobitz I (Wenkebach): PR interval gets longer till QRS dropped; reproduced with vagal stimulation
- Mobitz II: PR interval constant; intermittent block + occasional non-conductant P wave; may be fixed – 2:1, 3:1, 4:1, etc.

Third degree (Figure 34.10c):

- AV dissociation
- Regular P waves and regular QRS complexes with no relationship to each other

Myocardial infarction (Figure 34.11)

ST elevation
T wave inversion
Loss of height in R waves
Pathological Q waves
Return of ST segment to isoelectric line

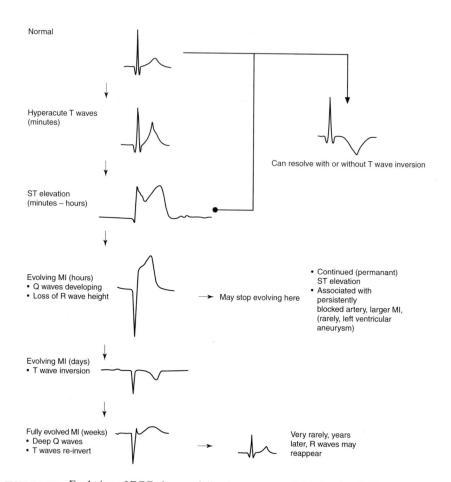

FIGURE 34.11 Evolution of ECG changes following a myocardial infarction (MI).

Bundle branch block

Widened QRS complexes (>0.12 s)

Record a 12-lead ECG

Introduce yourself. Explain what you are going to do: 'This machine will read the electrical activity of your heart and show me if anything is wrong. There is no pain and it cannot send any electricity out towards you'.

Invite any questions the patient might have. State that the patient may request a chaperone, if necessary.

Expose the patient from the waist up, as well as their ankles. Have them sitting up on a couch at 45°.

If a male patient has a hairy chest, state that you could shave parts of the chest, with the patient's permission, in order to minimize impedance.

Place 10 adhesive pads for the chest and limb leads (see below).

Chest leads (Figure 34.12)

V1: fourth intercostal space at right sternal edge
V2: fourth intercostal space at left sternal edge
V3: midway between V2 and V4
V4: over the apex, which is usually located in the fifth intercostal space in the left midclavicular line
V5: in the same horizontal line as V4 in the left anterior axillary line
V6: in the same horizontal line as V4 and V5 in the left midaxillary line

*Limb leads**

Red: right upper arm
Yellow: left upper arm
Green: left leg/pelvis
Black (earth): right leg/pelvis

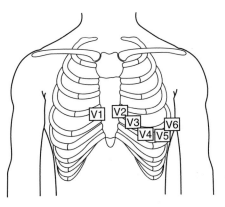

FIGURE 34.12 Placement of ECG electrodes.

*A useful tip is to remember the phrase 'Ride Your Green Bike', where the first letter of each word corresponds to the colours Red, Yellow, Green and Black. These create a 'circuit' starting at the patient's right arm and moving clockwise through to the right leg.

Attach the electrodes (which are labelled) to the appropriate pad. Ask the patient to remain still, breathe normally and not to talk for a few moments.

Turn the machine on and press 'Analyse'. Check the printout; if you do not have a good reading from all leads, check that all pads and electrodes are still attached firmly in the correct positions. Try again.

Once you have confirmed a clear ECG readout, label it with the patient's name and date of birth or hospital number, and time and date. It is also salient in clinical practice to state whether or not the patient is having 'Chest pain' or 'No chest pain'.

Thank the patient and offer to help them get dressed. Tell them you will now interpret their ECG recording and discuss it with the examiner.

Suggestions

Familiarize yourself with the equipment in any hospital ward. Medical wards, coronary care units (CCUs) and cardiovascular outpatient departments (OPDs) may be better places in which to practise recording than a busy A&E department.

35 Body mass index (BMI)

Scenario 1

You are the PRHO in General Practice. Mr Jeremy Golightly, a 54-year-old publican with type 2 diabetes, has come to have his BMI assessed. He weighs 107.2 kg and his height is 1.75 metres. Please advise him.

The body mass index (BMI) is a measure of a patient's weight relative to their height. Whilst this is useful in detecting obesity, bear in mind the pitfall of telling a very fit rugby forward or bodybuilder that they are obese, as they will have a raised BMI.

- Introduce yourself and explain what you would like to do.
- Gain consent.
- Ask the patient to remove their shoes.
- State that you would ideally ask the patient to strip to their underwear but for the sake of modesty, you will ask them to remove any heavy items of clothing (e.g. coats).
- Weight the patient in kilograms (kg).
- Measure the patient's height (m) – shoes still off.
- Offer to help the patient get dressed.

Using a calculator, find the BMI with the following formula:

$$BMI = weight/height^2 \qquad (kg/m^2)$$

Inform the patient, sensitively, of the significance of their measurement (Table 35.1). Advise the patient as to how they can improve their health. Remember to

TABLE 35.1   BMI values

Value (kg/m²)	Interpretation
<17	Consider anorexia
18–20	Low normal
20–25	Normal
25–30	Grade 1 (mild) obesity
30–40	Grade 2 (moderate) obesity
>40	Grade 3 (severe) obesity

reinforce that weight loss should be gradual and not rapid, which usually results in loss of lean body mass and not fat.

State that you would refer the patient to a dietician.

Lifestyle advice includes a couple of brief questions about heart disease, blood pressure and risk factors for coronary heart disease. This need not take more than a couple of minutes. Be aware that this station can be coupled with counselling about health, lifestyle and (for example) cardiovascular risk factors. Be guided by how much time you are given.

Arterial blood gases (oxygen therapy)

This common OSCE station can test clinical skills, understanding and interpretation of blood gases and even communication skills.

Notes to remember

- Venturi mask attachments work on all masks and control the exact amount of inspired oxygen (between 24% and 60%). Each attachment has a specific flow rate written on its side. Remember to adjust the oxygen flow rate to match the venturi fitting.
- A standard oxygen mask will deliver 50% at highest rates of flow.

(a)

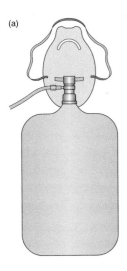

(b)

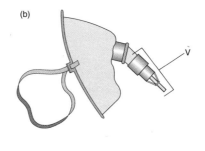

FIGURE 36.1   Oxygen masks. (a) Hudson mask with reservoir bag. (b) Venturi mask. **V**, the Venturi fitting is available in different colours, corresponding to different oxygen concentrations.

- Concentrations of up to 85% can be achieved using a non-rebreathe reservoir mask with oxygen flow rates of 10–15 l/min.

Interpretation of arterial blood gases (ABGs)

Normal ranges:

- pH: 7.35–7.45
- pCO_2: 4.7–6.0 kPa
- pO_2: >10.6 kPa
- HCO_3^- : 22–26 mmol/l

Three questions need to be asked:

1. What is the inspired concentration of O_2 (FiO_2)?
2. What are the pO_2 and pCO_2?
3. What are the pH and bicarbonate (HCO_3^-)?

For the following reasons:

1. High FiO_2 should raise the pO_2, such that a patient who would be hypoxic on air can have a pO_2 of >20. Knowing the patient is on oxygen will explain such readings.
2. These can tell us if there is respiratory disease:
   - $\downarrow pO_2$ and $\downarrow$/normal pCO_2 – type I respiratory failure; this is due to a ventilation/perfusion mismatch, found in asthma, PE, fibrosis and many other conditions
   - $\downarrow pO_2$ and $\uparrow pCO_2$ – type II respiratory failure; this is due to ventilatory failure, due to chronic hypoventilation, which can be physical (kyphosis) or neuromuscular in aetiology.
3. These can tell us if there is an acid–base disorder:
   - Acidosis ($\downarrow$pH) with
     - $\uparrow CO_2$ = respiratory acidosis (plus compensatory $\uparrow HCO_3^-$)
     - $\downarrow HCO_3^-$ = metabolic acidosis (plus $\downarrow CO_2$)
   - Alkalosis ($\uparrow$pH) with
     - $\downarrow CO_2$ = respiratory alkalosis (plus $\downarrow HCO_3^-$)
     - $\uparrow HCO_3^-$ = metabolic alkalosis (plus $\uparrow CO_2$)

Stations

In a typical station, you could well be introduced to a role player who is a breathless patient, aged 68 with known COPD.

- Introduce yourself.
- Ask the patient's name and age.
- Ask for a set of observations to be recorded on the patient, with emphasis on the oxygen saturations. If you do this, make sure there is no nail varnish on the finger you choose. The reading will come back low (below 92%).
- Put the patient on 24% oxygen immediately; explain this will help them breathe more easily.

Take a short history

Presenting complaint

Why have they come to hospital?

History of presenting complaint

Get a specific respiratory history: do they have any known lung disease, such as asthma, bronchitis or emphysema?
How severe is this problem? Any cough, sputum production (if so, what colour is it?), orthopnoea or paroxysmal nocturnal dyspnoea (PND)?
What is their current exercise tolerance? What is it normally?
Have they felt this way before? Were they hospitalized?

Drug history

Do they take any medicines? Specifically, inhalers, nebulizers, steroids?

Social history

Do/did they smoke? Or live with a smoker?
What is their job?

ABG results and oxygen therapy

Now that the patient is on oxygen, you would like to check the ABGs. Tell the examiner this; they pass you the following results:

pO_2	8.23
pCO_2	5.7

'This patient is hypoxic on 24% O_2 and has a normal pCO_2. Therefore he is in type I respiratory failure. I would like to administer some nebulized salbutamol and increase the concentration of inspired oxygen. I will check the blood gases again after this.'

Administer the salbutamol through a nebulizer, change the Venturi adaptor to
  35%.

The examiner hands you another set of results:

pO_2 14.0
pCO_2 6.4

'This patient's hypoxia has been corrected by inspired oxygen and nebulized
  salbutamol. However, they are now retaining CO_2, so I would choose to
  decrease the amount of inspired oxygen to 28%. I will check the blood
  gases again after this.'

State that this patient would benefit from antibiotics and a short course of
  steroid therapy. State you would also like to check the patient's PEFR and
  request a CXR.

Thank the patient.

Another station you may presented with is a young patient with a flare-up of
asthma. The management is sufficiently similar, although a high pCO_2 may
suggest that they are beginning to become exhausted and retain CO_2, and you
would indicate that senior help may be required.

37 Blood transfusion

It is tempting to think that transfusions are an easy and simple answer to patients with anaemia, that you can use blood for simply 'topping up' a patient's haemoglobin. This is far from the case. Blood supplies are not inexhaustible and there are inherent dangers, so you must use your ability to prescribe such products with thought and with caution.

A typical OSCE case will test your knowledge of the entire transfusion process. For instance: 'Mr Jackson is due to have an elective total hip replacement tomorrow, please Group and Save and/or set up a blood transfusion for him'.

Communication

This will involve introducing yourself to the patient, explaining what you are intending to do and why, then venesecting the patient (or fake arm).

1. You are going to take blood.
2. This blood is going to be stored in the blood lab.
3. It is going to be **grouped** – 'So we know what blood type you are'.
4. It will also be *screened* for 'atypical antibodies': 'These are rare proteins, which if present mean we have to use blood from which normal proteins are removed'.
5. It will also be **saved** – 'So we can arrange for blood to be provided urgently if necessary' (cross-matching).
6. 'For this operation, we are hoping not to have to give you any blood. However, should you lose a lot of blood we will have the opportunity to replace it sooner rather than later.'

7. 'Do you understand what I have just told you?'
8. 'Do you have any concerns or questions?' *Note that autologous blood can be used if the patient has beliefs that prevent them accepting a blood transfusion.*

Skills

Taking blood and filling out a blood form

Now you must gather your equipment:

- A tourniquet
- Alcohol wipes
- Vacutainer and needle
- A **Group and Save** bottle and form*
- Some gauze or cotton wool
- A pair of gloves

Once you have consent, make sure you have the correct patient. Refer to the notes for the patient's *full name, date of birth* and *hospital/unit number*. At the bedside, double-check this with the patient's wristband, which should have the same three pieces of information. If *any* of these identifiers differ, do not continue as you may have the wrong patient. You must ensure you have the correct information at hand before proceeding.

Assuming the information is all correct, you may proceed and bleed the patient. Make a point of filling out the information on the form and the bottle whilst still at the bedside after you have blood in the bottle. The point of all this is that giving the wrong blood to the wrong patient can kill (e.g. giving type A blood to a person with type O blood – *see later*), so we do not take any chances with mislabelling a bottle.

Cannulating and setting up a transfusion

If given a choice of cannulae, go for a *green* (18 G). Smaller bores are not suitable for transfusing blood as they are more likely to block if blood coagulates.

---

*Note that the colour and design of the bottle and form vary from trust to trust (generally pink-topped). There will inevitably be a choice and a chart showing what different bottles are used for. Do not be fazed, just look for the words 'Group and Save' – the process is designed to be simple.

1. Insert your cannula and check it is patent with a saline flush. Secure it in place.
2. Check the general state of the patient: 'Nurse, could you please perform a set of pre-transfusion observations?'.
3. Write up each unit of blood separately on the fluids section of the drug chart (Table 37.1).
4. Select a giving set, the dual-chamber variety.
5. Take the unit of blood, again checking that the information written on the bag, on the attached sheet of paper (the *compatibility form*) and the patient's wristband all agree.
6. Making sure it is locked, set the giving set up to the bag of blood.
   - Fill the first chamber completely.
   - Fill the second chamber halfway.
7. Run the giving set through, ensuring there are no air bubbles to be seen.
8. Attach the giving set to the cannula and let it run, stating that you would vary the drip rate to ensure the blood goes in at the correct rate.
9. 'I would now observe the patient for a few minutes in case he or she has an *acute haemolytic reaction.'**
10. 'I will also request that a nurse performs a set of observations in *15 minutes'* time.'
11. 'Should there be any sudden change in the patient's observations, or should the patient begin to feel toxic, I will *immediately stop the transfusion.'*
12. 'I would then *thoroughly examine the patient* in order to search for a cause, and manage the patient accordingly.'

TABLE 37.1   Example of writing up the fluid section of the drug chart

Date	Time	Fluid	Vol	Drug added	Dose	Duration
18/04	1700	Red cells 'Blood'	1U			3 h
18/04	2000	Red cells 'Blood'	1U	Furosemide*	20 mg	3 h

*Note that furosemide is commonly given with each second unit of blood to help maintain haemodynamic stability, thus avoiding CCF.

*The result of acute intravascular haemolysis of transfused red cells; this is a rare but potentially lethal complication of transfusion. Most often it is associated with ABO incompatibility, such as giving blood group A to a patient with blood group O. It is characterized by dyspnoea, fever, hypotension, chest pain and haemoglobinuria, and occurs rapidly after the onset of infusion. Complications are serious, including ARF and DIC.

13. Document in the notes what you have done, and why:

18/04 PRHO 1700

Blood results – 2 days post THR

Hb 7.9

WCC 5.2

Plt 310

<u>O/E</u> Patient is clinically anaemic; c/o dizziness.

P/ 80reg, HS/I + II + °, RS/NAD, Abdo/Soft, non-tender, +BS, PR-NAD

No evidence of occult bleeding. Pt not on NSAIDs.

Pre-op Hb 12.5.

<u>Plan</u>: 2U blood tonight. Review mané.

PRHO Blp 123

In NHS hospitals, these devices are typically those made by Graseby (Figure 38.1). There is the larger model, e.g. the 3100, and smaller syringe drivers, e.g. MS16A. Whilst the larger model is what you can expect in finals, familiarize yourself with both.

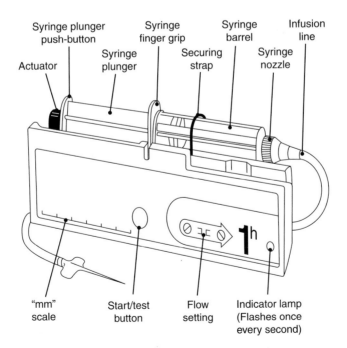

Syringe plunger push-button

Syringe finger grip

Syringe barrel

Infusion line

Syringe plunger

Securing strap

Syringe nozzle

Actuator

"mm" scale

Start/test button

Flow setting

Indicator lamp (Flashes once every second)

FIGURE 38.1 Syringe driver (Graseby MS16A).

Syringe pump

It is important to commandeer a syringe pump for practice prior to finals. Asking an experienced ITU nurse to show you how to use one is also paramount. This is a skill which, above all else, requires familiarity with the equipment.

Example: 'Please set up a 50 U Actrapid infusion for Mr Bloggs'.

1. State that you would look at the patient's notes and his recent BM (capillary glucose) readings.
2. Explain the procedure to the patient (if he is conscious) and invite questions.
3. Ensure IV access is available and patent.
4. Gather your equipment:
   - 50 U or 100 U syringe (in this case 50 U) – both have orange caps
   - 50 ml syringe with Luer lock (a screw at the top of the syringe)
   - Syringe pump and stand
   - Bag of normal saline
   - Bottle of Actrapid insulin
   - Line
   - Gloves
   - Stickers
5. Wash your hands and glove up.
6. Bring out the insulin slowly – do not wipe the top of the bottle.
7. Draw up 50 ml normal saline in your syringe.
8. Discard 0.5 ml of saline.
9. Add 50 U insulin (0.5 ml). **Note: You now have 50 U/50 ml of Actrapid = 1 U/ml.**
10. Add 5 ml air and gently roll syringe between your hands (as if you were starting a camp fire) to mix it.
11. Discard the air and run through (prime) the line.
12. Attach the syringe to the pump, noting that it sits in the recess under the retaining clamp. Ensure the ear of the syringe is located in the syringe barrel slot. Secure the plunger in the slot of the actuator.
13. Purge the pump (by pressing the 'Purge' button). This takes up the mechanical slack and ensures that administration of the drug commences when the 'Start' button is pressed (later).
14. Attach the line to the patient.
15. Find two stickers (see Figure 38.2) and fill in the relevant information. Attach one to the syringe and one to the line.
16. Set rate of infusion in ml/hour on the pump (which, because of the concentration you prepared, is now also units/hour)

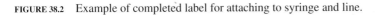

DRUGS ADDED TO THIS INFUSION				
PATIENT Joe Bloggs			WARD Paget	
DRUG Actrapid 50iu/50mls =1iu/ml DILUENT N/Saline	AMOUNT 50ml	BATCH No 6		PREP'D BY to CHECKED BY Sup
DATE PREP'D 7/2/.04 TIME PREP'D 1500	EXP. DATE 5/5/05 EXP. TIME 0900		ROUTE IV	
DISCONTINUE IF CLOUDINESS OR PRECIPITATE DEVELOPS				

FIGURE 38.2   Example of completed label for attaching to syringe and line.

17. Press 'Start'.
18. Wait a few minutes to check that no problems arise.
19. Document what you have done in the notes.
20. Ask the nurse to do regular blood glucose measurements on the patient.
21. Inform staff that no patient or relative must use a mobile phone near the pump, as this can interfere with its functioning.

Notes

● If the alarm goes off, check to see if there is an occlusion in the line or at the site of access.
● Also check the rate is correct (the pump will alarm if a very high rate is set), syringe is correct type and how much solution is left (the pump usually gives a three-minute warning when the solution runs out).
● Insulin denatures plastic, so state that the line must be changed every 24 hours.
● If you are asked to prescribe morphine for a PCA (patient-controlled analgesia), which uses the same pumps, use sterile water as a dilutent, not saline.
● If prescribing morphine, consider locking the device under a protective cover.

Syringe drivers

● Smaller than the pumps, these are often portable devices, used to deliver a variety of drugs (heparin, insulin, morphine, etc.) via a subcutaneous route.
● Rates of fluid delivery are calculated in *mm of travel per hour*, not ml/hour. It has a minimum rate of 1 mm/hour and a maximum of 99 mm/hour.

- The largest syringe the driver can take is usually 35 ml but it can take any brand.
- Fluid length is measured *after* priming the line. Calculate using the following formula:

$$\frac{\text{Fluid length (mm)}}{\text{Required infusion period (hours)}}$$

- Use a paperclip to set the rate.
- Secure syringe to driver using the strap.
- Press the white actuator button, which will lock the plunger.
- Insert battery and press 'Start'.

Male catheterization

Rest assured that this will be performed on a mannequin, but you must assume that there is a conscious patient who may want some information about what you are going to do.

- Introduce yourself.
- Explain what you intend to do and why (for prostatism, 'We can help relieve pain and discomfort by emptying your bladder'; for renal failure, 'It is very important that we measure exactly how much fluid is going in and out of you, I do hope you appreciate that').
- Reassure the patient by telling him you will be using a local anaesthetic so he shouldn't feel too much discomfort.
- State that you would request an assistant, and a chaperone if necessary.

Gather your equipment:

- Trolley
- 14–16 G French Foley catheter
- Lignocaine gel
- 10 ml sterile water
- 10 ml syringe
- Catheter pack: consists of a kidney dish, sterile gloves, drape, gauze, a pot and a rubbish bag
- Antiseptic solution
- Catheter bag

Close the curtains

- Position the patient supine with his genitalia and abdomen fully exposed.

- State that if the patient had a foreskin, you would ask him to retract it.
- Wash your hands.

From this point onwards, pay special attention to maintaining your sterile field. Should you lose it, it is important to recognize this and point it out. State that you would, under normal circumstances, begin again. The kindly examiner should appreciate that you have pointed this out and ask you to continue anyway.
  Open your catheter pack on to the trolley.

- Open out on to the sterile area: catheter (has a sleeve), lignocaine gel, syringe, sterile gloves.
- Pour the antiseptic solution into the pot.
- Open the catheter bag. Position at the foot of the bed for the moment.
- Put your sterile gloves on.
- Attach the rubbish bag to the side of the trolley.
- Open the catheter out.
- Ask the assistant (examiner) to open your sterile water, making sure you both check that it *is* what you think and has not passed its expiry date. They can hold the ampule, whilst you withdraw the water, maintaining your sterile field. Put the syringe back on the field.
- Drape the patient, by tearing a hole through which his penis will fit.
- Use your non-dominant hand to hold the penis with a piece of gauze.
- Soak the remaining pieces of gauze in the pot and wipe the head of the penis, heading away from the urethra once with each piece of gauze.
- Holding the penis at 90° to the patient, inject the lignocaine gel, keeping an eye on the patient.
- State that you would normally give the anaesthetic five minutes to work.
- Remove the pot from the kidney dish and place it between the patient's legs so you can catch any urine when it begins to flow.
- Take your catheter and make sure that all of it remains within the sterile field, which still includes the drape and the kidney dish (where the distal end should sit).
- Gently advance it through the urethra, keeping an eye on the patient for any signs of pain or discomfort.
- If you meet resistance, position the penis more caudally (i.e. nearer its normal position) and try again.
- Once you are in far enough, urine should pass into the kidney dish.
- Use the syringe to gently inflate the balloon, keeping a constant eye on the patient.*

*Inflating the balloon whilst in the prostate will result in pain and damage, so you must be careful.

- Attach the catheter bag.
- Gently retract the catheter until a resistance is felt.
- Reposition the foreskin and discard all of your rubbish.
- Remove your gloves, wash your hands and thank the patient.
- Ask the nurse to record the urine output from this patient.
- Document the procedure including your details, date and time, whether urine was drained, how much was drained, and whether it was stained with blood, as well as the type and size of catheter, and that aseptic technique was used.

40 Venous cannulation and setting up a drip

Introduce yourself and gain consent.
  Gather your equipment:

- 20 G cannula (typically coloured pink) should suffice for IV fluids in an adult
- Tourniquet
- Cannula dressing
- Giving set
- Three alcohol swabs
- Gloves
- Bag of fluid (i.e. 1 litre 0.9% saline)
- Sharps box

Proceed with the cannulation:

- Check the contents of the bag and its expiry date. Ask the examiner to countercheck these facts.
- Run the giving set through and 'clamp' it, ensuring there are no air bubbles in the tubing.
- Look for a suitable vein; likely spots are in the antecubital fossa and dorsum of the hand.
- Apply the tourniquet and re-check for the vein.
- Don your gloves.
- Clean the site over the vein once with each swab.
- Remove the cannula from the pack and remove the sheath.
- Stretch the skin over the vein, which should secure the vein.
- Insert the needle at an angle of around 30° to the skin, with the bevel up.
- When you successfully see blood flushing into the hub, advance the cannula without the needle.

- Release the tourniquet with gentle pressure over the vein.
- Remove the needle and discard it safely in the sharp bin.
- Attach the giving set.
- Fix the cannula and the tubing securely.
- Adjust the drip to run, watching that it is working successfully.

Notes

When asked what size cannula you would use, ask the examiner what the situation at hand is.

- Surgical emergencies (i.e. perforations) require the largest possible bore – grey (16 G) or larger.
- Blood transfusions – green (18 G).
- Maintenance IV fluids in a patient who is not in shock – pink (20 G).
- Difficult veins, slow IV fluids or IV medications in a patient who can take fluids orally – blue (22 G).

41

Nasogastric intubation

This is an important procedure that *House Officers* are asked to perform, needed before and after GI surgery, in cases of poisoning or when there is a serious risk of aspiration in the patient.

Introduce yourself and explain what you would like to do and gain consent for the procedure. Gather your equipment:

- 16 F Ryle's tube
- Xylocaine spray
- KY jelly
- Glass of water

Proceed with the intubation:

- Sit the patient up.
- Wash your hands and don a pair of non-sterile gloves.
- Measure the distance from the tip of the nose to the xiphisternum via an ear lobe. This will correspond to the distance you will need to advance your tube to reach the stomach. Most tubes are marked for measurement, so keep a note of the required distance.
- Spray the chosen nostril with xylocaine spray.
- Cover the end of the tube with KY jelly.
- Pass the tube into the nostril along the floor of the nose into the nasopharynx, aiming towards the occiput.
- Ask the patient to take sips of water and advance the tube as they sip (thus ensuring the epiglottis is closed).
- Advance the tube to the predetermined distance; if you are in the correct place, you should not meet with much resistance.

- Inject a small amount of air into the tube and listen over the xiphisternum and left hypochondrium for sounds of 'bubbling'. Alternatively you can aspirate some fluid and test with litmus paper that it is hydrochloric acid.
- Tape the tube to the patient's nose.
- State that you could check a nasogastric tube was in situ with the aid of a CXR.
- Document the procedure including your name and bleep, date and time, whether any fluid was drained.

42

Public health and evidence-based medicine

'The science and art of promoting health, preventing disease, and prolonging life through the organized efforts of society.'*

It is easy to overlook public health as an important aspect of modern medicine. This is unfortunate. Consider conditions with national screening in place where reliable tests can save lives. Also consider that public health is a *major* part of undergraduate and postgraduate exams.

This chapter has been divided into three sections:

- Diagnostic tests and screening
- Types of study
- Departments and public health bodies

Diagnostic tests and screening

You will be familiar with Table 42.1, where a given diagnostic test is compared with the presence of disease (as demonstrated by a 'gold standard' test). In reality, we rarely have proof of disease, just a high index of suspicion. As such, we are actually comparing a diagnostic test with the 'gold standard'.[†]

Remember:

- sen*s*itivity measures *s*ickness
- speci*f*icity measures *f*itness.

*Acheson D. Independent Inquiry into Inequalities in Health. HMSO, London, 1988.
[†]Examples include venography for DVT and histology for cancer.

TABLE 42.1

| | | True result (gold standard) | | |
		Positive	*Negative*	
Test result	Positive	a (TP)	b (FP)	PPV
	Negative	c (FN)	d (TN)	NPV
		Sensitivity	Specificity	

TP, true positive; FP, false positive; FN, false negative; TN, true negative.

Sensitivity (a/[a+c] or TP/[TP+FN]) – the proportion of persons with disease who are correctly identified by a screening test or case definition as having disease. Thus, the proportion of true positives. (Sensitivity measures *sickness*.)

Specificity (d/[b+d] or TN/[FP+TN]) – the proportion of persons without disease who are correctly identified by a screening test or case definition as not having disease. Thus, the proportion of true negatives. (Speci*f*icity measures *f*itness.)

Positive predictive value (a/[a+b] or TP/[TP+FP]) – the proportion of persons with a positive test result who are truly positive.

Negative predictive value (d/(c+d) or TN/(FN+TN)) – the proportion of persons with a negative test result who are truly negative.

A valid test relies on having a high sensitivity and specificity. In reality, one decreases as the other increases so a balance must be struck between them.

Consider what each of these definitions really means:

- If *sensitivity* is low, there exist a lot of FNs (c) who will carry on life without treatment and may suffer from the disease.
- If *specificity* is low, there exist a lot of FPs (b) who will go through investigations and treatments they do not need.
- *PPV* holds the true value for the patient. Should you test positive, this equates to the chance that you really have the disease.
- *NPV* meanwhile serves to reassure. Should you test negative, this will be the chance that you really do not have the disease.

The four definitions above are mandatory core knowledge – learn them.
Consider DVTs:

- D-dimers have high NPV – with so many positive tests, it is negative tests that are significant. So, not good for finding a DVT but great for excluding one.
- Venography is the *gold standard* (a or TP is very high). Hence, it will have a high sensitivity and PPV. Good for finding disease – if test is positive you probably do have DVT.

Screening can be defined as 'any medical investigation that does not arise from a patient's request for advice for a specific complaint'.

Conditions with national screening programmes

- Phenylketonuria
- Congenital hypothyroid (TSH at birth)
- Breast cancer
- Cervical cancer

Why do we screen? How do we know what to screen for? And how best to do this? There are specific criteria for implementing a national screening programme.

The condition

- Important health burden
- Epidemiology and natural history understood (from risk factor to development to declared disease)
- Primary prevention interventions already implemented

The test

- Simple, safe, precise and validated
- Agreed policy of further diagnostic investigations

The treatment

- Effective treatment available and evidence that early treatment has better outcome than late treatment
- Agreed policies as to who gets treated and how

The screening programme

- Evidence from randomized controlled study that programme is effective in reducing mortality or morbidity
- Entire programme (test through to treatment) is acceptable to healthcare professionals and public, clinically, socially and ethically
- Benefit should outweigh physical and psychological harm
- Opportunity cost economically balanced in relation to expenditure on medical care
- All other options for managing the condition have been fully considered

The Bradford Hill criteria

These criteria for causation were developed for use in occupational medicine but have been widely applied in other fields. The key criteria required to establish causation are commonly:

- *temporal relationship*: obviously the alleged causative agent must precede the disease. In addition, if it is possible to show a temporal relationship, as between exposure to the factor in the population and frequency of the disease, the case is strengthened.
- *specificity*: if the determinant being studied can be isolated from others and shown to produce changes in the incidence of the disease, e.g. if thyroid cancer can be shown to have a higher incidence specifically associated with fluoride, this is convincing evidence of causation.
- *biological plausibility*.
- *coherence*.

Types of study

Cross-sectional study

A representative sample of people are interviewed, examined or otherwise studied using data collected at a single time to provide a 'snapshot' of information. Good for working out prevalence.

Cohort study

A research study, in which group(s) of people identified by certain characteristics or statistical factors, such as age, are followed and observed over a long period of time. A typical study may involve recruiting an initially healthy group (cohort) of people exposed to different levels (or not at all) of a particular risk factor (e.g. cigarette smoke) for a disease (e.g. lung cancer). The participants are followed up for a number of years to compare how many in each group develop a particular disease or other outcome. It is good for incidence of common diseases and gives a relative risk.

Case control study

This is good for rare diseases (MND, MS, etc.) and gives an odds ratio. For example, regarding lung cancer and smoking, smokers are three times more likely to develop cancer. It is susceptible to bias, e.g. patients with cancer sometimes underestimate the amount they have smoked and patients without tend to exaggerate.

Ecological study

Information is gained at the ecological level (cheap) by comparing populations in different geographical locations. For example, one may look at pollution levels in different countries and compare the prevalence of asthma.

Meta-analysis

The statistical analysis of data taken from a number of similar research studies on a specific topic. The aim is to integrate the findings and pool the data to identify the overall trends of the response.

Migrant study

For example, the effect of a Western diet on immigrants from non-Western countries.

Audit

A process that involves the examination or review of practices, processes or performances in a systematic way to establish the extent to which they meet predetermined criteria. The procedure includes identifying problems, developing solutions, making changes to practice, then reviewing the whole operation or service again. The whole process is called an audit 'cycle'.

Randomized controlled trials

Studies in which participants are randomly allocated to either a treatment (or other intervention, such as screening) group or a control group that doesn't receive the treatment or intervention. Both groups are followed up for a specific period. The outcomes, which are specified at the outset (e.g. weight loss, reduction in heart attacks), are measured to determine any difference between the two groups.

Departments and public health bodies

Cochrane collaboration

This is an international network of nine research centres, of which the UK Cochrane Centre is a member. Its function is to develop, maintain and disseminate up-to-date information from systematic reviews of healthcare trials. The main output of the collaboration is the Cochrane Library. The Cochrane Centre coordinates randomized controlled trials to produce the Cochrane database (a summary and meta-analysis of RCTs). It tends to focus on clinical outcomes.

National Institute for Clinical Excellence (NICE)

NICE assesses the effectiveness of new (and existing) treatments and diagnostic tests. It produces and disseminates clinical guidelines to promote cost-effective therapies and uniform clinical standards. It gives guidance on health technologies, clinical managements of specific conditions and referrals from primary to secondary care.*

Department of Health (DoH)

The Department of Health is divided into a policy (thinking) arm and an executive (NHS – doing) arm. The 'doing' arm is divided into regional health authorities, which comprise local authorities, strategic health authorities and primary care trusts.

Strategic health authority (SHAs)

In 2002, England's 95 health authorities were replaced by 28 larger health authorities, each covering an average of 1.5 million people. Many of their former responsibilities were passed on to primary care trusts and they now have a more strategic function. SHAs manage the NHS locally and are a key link between the Department of Health and the NHS. They also ensure that national priorities (such as programmes for improving cancer services) are integrated into plans for the local health service. They are responsible for developing strategies, ensuring high-quality performance and building capacity in the local health service.

Primary care trusts (PCTs)

Responsible for the planning and commissioning of health services for their local population. For example, PCTs must make sure there are enough GPs to serve the community and that they are accessible to patients. PCTs must also

*Coales U. *Get through MRCGP: Oral and Video Modules.* RSM Press, London, 2004, pp. 52–3.

guarantee the provision of other health services including hospitals, dentists, mental healthcare, walk-in centres, NHS Direct, patient transport (including A&E), population screening, pharmacies and opticians. In addition, they are responsible for integrating health and social care so the two systems work together for patients.

General Medical Council (GMC)

All doctors practising in the UK are required to be registered with the GMC, on the General Medical Register. The GMC requires doctors to subscribe to a set of ethical standards and hence it polices the profession. Its ultimate sanction is erasure from the Register and/or referral to the civil authorities.

Clinical governance

There are many definitions for this. One succinct example we found was: 'Clinical governance is the initiative of the White Paper, *The New NHS: modern, dependable*. It is a framework to improve patient care through high standards. It promotes personal and team development, cost-effective, evidence-based clinical practice, risk avoidance, and the investigation of adverse situations'.* The most succinct example is 'the modification of healthcare systems to optimise patient care'.†

The Commission for Health Improvement (CHI) oversees the quality of clinical governance and of services. It reviews all types of organizations, including PCTs, hospitals and general practices for quality of services to patients.

---

*Coales U. *Get through MRCGP: Oral and Video Modules*. RSM Press, London, 2004, pp. 52–3.
†De Halpert P, Pollock I, Lynch J, Beatrie M, *Basic Child Health Practice Papers*, Pastest, 2004, p. 119.

Index

T

tamponade 237
tap test 90
tension pneumothorax 237
teratogenesis, warfarin 76
thromboembolism 237
thumb, Z deformity 148
thyroid examination 171–73
Tinel's test 148, 150
tone, upper limb 137–8, 141–2, 150–1
tongue examination 119
tongue movements 120
Trendelenburg's test 90–1, 159–60
tricuspid regurgitation 99, 101,
    102
tricuspid stenosis 99
trigeminal nerve
    facial examination 118
    motor function 118
    tests 109–11
trochlear nerve
    IVth nerve palsy 112–13
    tests 110
Ts, four 237
tuberculosis, AFB test 108

U

ulnar neuropathy 147
upper limb examination 141–8
    drift 142
upper motor neurone lesions 138

V

vaginal examination 193–7
vagus nerve tests 109–10, 119
varicose veins 32, 89–91
veins, Trendelenburg's test 90–1
venous cannulation 281–3
venous pulses, jugular 98–9
ventricular fibrillation 257–8
    DC defibrillation 235–7
ventricular septal defect 218
ventricular tachycardia 258
    pulseless VT 235
Venturi (oxygen) mask 266
vestibulocochlear nerve tests 110
Virchow's node 82
visual acuity 111
visual fields
    confrontational 114
    defects 115
vitamin K 78
VIth nerve palsy 112, 113
vomiting, paediatrics 215

W

warfarin 76–7
Weber's test 119, 132
wheezing 72–3
written exams 6

Z

Z deformity, thumb 148